NEUROENDOCRINE TUMORS

A COMPREHENSIVE GUIDE TO DIAGNOSIS AND MANAGEMENT

FIFTH EDITION

Updated with ICD-10 Codes

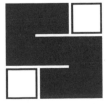

Eugene A. Woltering
Aaron I. Vinik
Thomas M. O'Dorisio
Vay Liang W. Go
Gregg Mamikunian

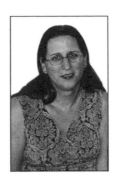

The fifth edition of the NET's handbook
is dedicated to Dr. Maria Tellez

Since Dr. Maria Tellez's arrival at Inter Science in 2003, she was chosen twice as "Employee of the Year" in 2007 and 2011. Her dedication, devotion and performance under the most demanding circumstances are beyond description. No words can describe my respect and admiration for her enormous scientific talents and immense personal integrity and humility.

How fortunate for Inter Science and its employees and associates to have the privilege of knowing and working with her. Thank you Maria.

Sincerely,

Gregg
August 27, 2012

Inter Science Institute's G.I. Council 2002-2012

Chairman

Eugene A. Woltering, M.D., F.A.C.S.

The James D. Rives Professor of Surgery and Neurosciences
Chief of the Sections of Surgical Endocrinology & Oncology
Director of Surgery Research
The Louisiana State University Health Sciences Center
New Orleans, LA 70112

Executive Members

Aaron I. Vinik, M.D., Ph.D., FCP., MACP

Professor of Medicine, Pathology and Neurobiology
Director of Strelitz Diabetes Research Center & Neuroendocrine Unit
Eastern Virginia Medical School
Norfolk, VA 23510

Thomas M. O'Dorisio, M.D.

Professor of Medicine
Director of Neuroendocrine Tumor Program
Clinical Attending, Holden Comprehensive Cancer Center
University of Iowa College of Medicine
Iowa City, IA 52242

Vay Liang W. (Bill) Go, M.D.

Distinguished Professor of Medicine
David Geffen School of Medicine at UCLA
University of California at Los Angeles
Los Angeles, CA 90095

Gregg Mamikunian, M.S.

Chief Executive Officer
Inter Science Institute, Inc.

In 1971, Inter Science Institute (ISI) established its first commercial GI laboratory, and six years later published the first GI handbook that listed critical GI peptides of clinical significance. The commercial availability of such tests was groundbreaking at that time. A few years later, more than twenty cases of Zollinger-Ellison Syndrome were documented surgically as a result of ISI's gastrin analyses. As a result of the chemical evidence of these hormone concentrations, many pancreatic, adrenal, ovarian, renal, and gastric tumors were determined at leading medical institutions.

It is no accident that the field of neuroendocrine laboratory procedures at ISI began to expand its menu, that was first available in 1994, to develop specific, additional biomarkers to assist in the diagnosis and treatment of neuroendocrine patients. In 2002, a decade ago, ISI established its second GI Council with the vision of presenting the medical community with advances in GI, pancreatic and regulatory peptides. Since then, we have published a dozen peer-reviewed scientific articles as to the utility, significance, and predictability of these biomarkers to provide diagnosis in healthy and disease states.

The history of any major discovery, not only in medical science, and whether accidental or intentional, has been amply directed towards the benefit of all mankind. It would be foolhardy for a university, government laboratory, or private research laboratory to lay claim as guarantors and guardians of such lofty ideals and goals. When any one of such entity waves the banner of exclusivity, it diminishes the noble pursuit of scientific inquiry and achievement. Fortunately, history can recite endlessly the great achievements, discoveries, and breakthroughs that have emerged through the collaborative efforts of educational, governmental and commercial entities.

ISI will, as it has in the past, expand its reach to academic and commercial institutions both in the US and overseas in the furtherance of neuroendocrine advances for the benefit of the patient.

Gregg Mamikunian
Chief Executive Officer
August 12, 2012

Acknowledgments to the Fifth Edition

A special appreciation and thank you to Dr. Aaron I. Vinik for his valuable time afforded in bridging the scientific content and clinical applications in this current edition.

The authors of the fifth edition of the neuroendocrine tumors handbook sincerely thank M. Sue O'Dorisio, M.D., Ph.D. for her contribution updating Chapter 2 of the handbook. Our thanks to Debra C. Godsey, R.N. for updating the ICD-9 codes throughout the various chapters.

A special and great thank you to Mia S. Tepper, MBA for the months of diligent attention to every detail in reviewing and editing this manuscript.

The fifth edition does reflect the dedication of the G.I. Council members' ever-ready guidance to ensure a handbook that reflects their commitment to excellence in providing current and credible scientific information to the physician, and the ultimate beneficiary ---- the patient.

To this end, my personal and sincere thanks to each of the Council members, Drs. Vinik, O'Dorisio, Go and its chairman, Dr. Woltering for a decade of selfless service, guidance and encouragement.

Thank you,
Gregg Mamikunian
Inter Science Institute 2012

ACKNOWLEDGMENTS TO THE FOURTH EDITION

The authors of the 4th edition of the *Neuroendocrine Tumors* handbook sincerely appreciate the contribution of M. Sue O'Dorisio, MD, PhD for the second chapter of the handbook. It is a great honor and privilege to have professor Sue O'Dorisio's hitherto unpublished chapter appear in the ISI Neuroendocrine book.

The GI Council welcomes professor Joy Ardill, MD, of Royal Victoria Hospital of Northern Ireland, (UK), for her scientific collaborative association with Inter Science Institute.

The Council acknowledges Donald W. Richardson, MD of Eastern Virginia Medical School (EVMS) for his contribution on sections of pituitary tumors, Cushings and diabetes insipidus.

Our thanks to Debbie Godsey for updating the ICD-9 codes throughout the chapters of the 3rd and 4th editions. Also, our thanks to Etta Vinik for her work on certain sections of the handbook.

A special thanks to Mia Tepper for the months of diligent attention to details in reviewing the manuscript.

The executive members of the council gratefully acknowledges the dedication, foresight and leadership of its chairman Eugene A. Woltering, MD.

The enormous contributions of Arthur A. Vinik, MD, Thomas M. O'Dorisio, MD, and Vay Liang W. (Bill) Go, MD, encompassing the scientific matrix and its accretion into a clinically useful and diagnostically relevant format must be applauded.

Gregg Mamikunian
Inter Science Institute 2009
Reprinted from Inter Science Institute's *Neuroendocrine Tumors: A Comprehensive Guide to Diagnosis and Management* handbook, 2009.

ACKNOWLEDGMENTS TO THE THIRD EDITION

The GI Council of Inter Science Institute presents this comprehensive guide to diagnosis and management of neuroendocrine tumors to provide information and inspiration to all levels of clinicians, from novices to those professionally engaged in the field of neuroendocrine research, treatment, and analyses. This guidebook adds the new dimension of patient monitoring, not only through powerfully discriminating assays but through the recognition of clinical presentations and syndromes. This expertise is made possible by more than 150 years of cumulative experience of the advisory council.

Since the publication of the first GI Handbook in 1977 up to the current edition of *Neuroendocrine Tumors*, Inter Science Institute has been at the forefront of bridging the gap between academic medicine and the availability of the most current tests for patient diagnosis. In the intervening three and a half decades, unparalleled progress has been made both in the diagnosis and treatment of gastrointestinal, pancreatic, and neuroendocrine tumors.

This book is meant to be a *beacon* not only for listing tests but for all aspects of neuroendocrine tumors. Its publication represents a move from static text to the modern era of communication which allows for dynamic, continuously updating links to the ISI website, interscienceinstitute.com, as well as endotext.com as reference sources. Additionally, the book combines several references from the previous edition with an updated bibliography, in recognition of past contributions to the present.

Special thanks to our dedicated reviewers of this publication, Etta J. Vinik and Mia S. Tepper.

Finally, my appreciation and thanks to professors Vinik, Woltering, O'Dorisio, and Go for imparting their knowledge to the synergistic confluence that has given birth to this unique edition. Thank you, Arthur, Gene, O'Do, and Bill.

Gregg Mamikunian
Inter Science Institute 2006
Reprinted from Inter Science Institute's *Neuroendocrine Tumors: A Comprehensive Guide to Diagnosis and Management* handbook, 2006.

Acknowledgments to the Second Edition

The current 1997 edition of the *GI, Pancreatic Hormones, Related Peptides and Compounds*® handbook presents comprehensive information for many rare procedures and tests that have been requested in the course of the past twenty-eight years.

The handbook reflects the tremendous advances that have been made since 1977. The number of tests offered has increased six-fold in addition to increasing specificity, sensitivity of antibodies, and purity of the standards. The protocols dealing with challenges and provocative testing has been expanded with the latest information. The section on the physiology of the GI and Pancreatic Hormones has been updated as an adjunct to the various procedures in the handbook.

Furthermore, the handbook covers a vast area of gastrointestinal, pancreatic, and other related procedures. Many of these procedures are clearly out of the realm of routine testing and request. On the other hand, quite a number of the procedures are indicators in the clinical confirmation of certain syndromes and disease states. Inter Science has witnessed the phenomenon over the years of the transformation of research-oriented procedures becoming useful, routine, and critical determining factors in the diagnosis and management of certain GI-related endocrinopathies.

A special acknowledgment to Alan C. Kacena for his dedication and service of twenty-five years at Inter Science Institute and in bringing the current edition of the GI Hormones handbook into reality.

Gregg Mamikunian
Inter Science Institute 1997
Reprinted from Inter Science Institute's *GI, Pancreatic Hormones, Related Peptides and Compounds*® handbook, 1997.

Acknowledgments to the First Edition

The great majority of the gastrointestinal and pancreatic peptide hormones and polypeptide assays listed in this handbook would not have been even remotely possible had it not been for the tremendous generosity and cooperation of all the individuals listed below. Without their assistance, the establishment of the GI Hormones Laboratory at Inter Science Institute would not have been a reality.

Inter Science Institute gratefully acknowledges and thanks Professor V. Mutt of GI Hormones Laboratory of Karolinska Institute (Sweden) for his immense assistance and encouragement; Professor N. Yanaihara (Japan); Dr I.M. Samloff (USA); Professor J.C. Brown (Canada); Dr R. Geiger (Germany); Dr R.E. Chance (USA); Professor A.G.E. Pearse (England); Dr J.E. Hall (England); Dr R.I. Harvey (England) and Professor M. Bodanszky (USA).

Our sincerest appreciation to Professor John H. Walsh of the University of California at Los Angeles for his collaboration over the many years and his review and many suggestions regarding this presentation.

Finally, a special acknowledgment to Dr Herbert Gottfried of Inter Science Institute for his long and dedicated years in bringing the GI Hormones Laboratory into fruition.

Gregg Mamikunian
Inter Science Institute 1997
Reprinted from Inter Science Institute's *GI & Pancreatic Hormones and Polypeptides®* handbook, 1977.

This book is designed as an educational tool, as well as a practical manual for the diagnosis of patients with suspected neuroendocrine tumors (NETs) and a variety of associated gastrointestinal disorders, guiding the physician to long-term follow-up. Conceptually, this handbook is more than a list of laboratory tests, as it comprises seven sections total including:

Chapter 1, Diagnosing and Treating GEP NETs describes the complexity of the problems involved with suspected NETs. It then simplifies the problems by viewing them under these headings: *Clinical presentation, What to look for, and Next Step* providing guidance throughout the decision-making process from diagnosis to follow-up. *Includes detailed tables with Syndrome Tumor Type, Sites, Hormones, and ICD-10 codes.*

Chapter 2, NETs in Children and Young Adults provides a discussion of non-familial neuroendocrine tumors children, young adults, and adults less than thirty years old.

Chapter 3, Clinical Presentations and their Syndromes highlights the clinical manifestations related to the neuroendocrine system for the many clinical manifestations associated with excessive peptide amine release and provides a step-by-step approach to possible diagnoses.

Chapter 4, Assays measure hormone excretion in healthy and disease states. Tests are listed alphabetically and are set out with clear and concise requirements, including: patient preparation; specimen collection, with preservative tube requirements (such as, G.I., Z-tube™, and TRH); important precautions; shipping instructions, and *CPT* codes.

Chapter 5, Profiles represent a collection of assays that should provide guidance to the diagnosing physician when ordering them as a profile. This section also includes the following: patient preparation, specimen collection, important precautions, shipping instructions, and *CPT* codes for insurance purposes.

Chapter 6, Dynamic Tests presents dynamic challenge and provocative protocols. The drug doses outlined in these tests are recommendations only and should be reviewed and confirmed by the attending physician on an individual patient basis. Dynamic challenge protocols can be dangerous and should be performed *only* under the direct and constant supervision of trained medical personnel, who are familiar with the "expected" and potentially "unexpected" responses to provocative testing.

Chapter 7, Algorithm for the Evaluation & Management of NETs presents a multitude of guidelines and suggested therapeutic algorithms adapted from the ISI G.I. Council, NANETS, ENETS, and NCCN.

Abbreviations are spelled out in the text the first time each is used. A list of abbreviations appears in the back of the text.

Appendix, Sample worksheets and ISI Test Requisition Slip provide a simple mechanism to order tests for a variety of syndromes and symptoms. Worksheet categories include recommendations for: radiology, routine labs, ISI lab tests, provocative testing, with CPT codes and updated with ICD-10 codes.

Index provides a comprehensive listing of the terminology and test names.

TABLE OF CONTENTS

TABLE OF CONTENTS

Chapter 5

TABLE OF CONTENTS

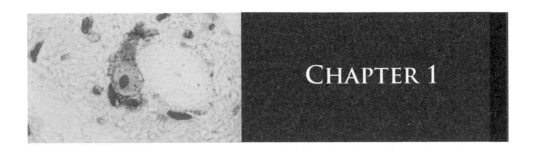

CHAPTER 1

DIAGNOSING AND TREATING GASTROENTEROPANCREATIC TUMORS, INCLUDING ICD-10 CODES

NEUROENDOCRINE TUMORS
A COMPREHENSIVE GUIDE TO DIAGNOSIS AND MANAGEMENT

GASTROENTEROPANCREATIC TUMORS

Endocrine tumors of the gastroenteropancreatic (GEP) axis (involving the gastrointestinal [GI] system, stomach, and pancreas) are comprised of cells capable of amine precursor uptake and decarboxylation, hence the prior name "APUDomas." The morphologic similarity of the APUD cells suggested a common embryologic origin, indicated by the term "protodifferentiated stem cell," now believed to derive from the endoderm and capable of giving rise to a variety of tumors **(Fig. 1-1)**.

Neuroendocrine tumors (NETs) are neoplasms that arise from cells of the endocrine (hormonal) and nervous systems. Many are benign, while some are malignant. NETs are rare and produce symptoms which are often difficult to distinguish from the symptoms of more common conditions, such as inflammatory bowel disease (IBD) or irritable bowel syndrome (IBS). Serum and plasma biomarkers are commonly utilized to diagnose NETs in patients with common gastrointestinal complaints.

- NETs share common features, such as looking similar, having special secretory granules, and often producing biogenic amines and polypeptide hormones.
- Arise from various neuroendocrine cells whose normal function is to serve as the neuroendocrine interface. Neuroendocrine cells are present not only in endocrine glands throughout the body that produce hormones, but also diffusely in all body tissues.
- Enterochromaffin cells, give rise to carcinoid tumors, were identified in 1897 by Kulchitsky and their secretion of serotonin established in 1953
- NETS were called APUDomas show amine precursor (L-DOPA and 5-hydroxytryptophan) uptake and decarboxylation to produce biogenic amines, such as catecholamines and serotonin.
- The current view is that neuroendocrine cells reside throughout the body in all tissues and can de-differentiate into tumor cells.
- NETs include:
    - tumors of the gastrointestinal tract
    - the pancreatic islet cells
    - thymus and lung tumors,
    - medullary carcinoma of the parafollicular cells of the thyroid.
    - Tumors in the pituitary, parathyroid, and adrenomedullary glands and paraganglion cells

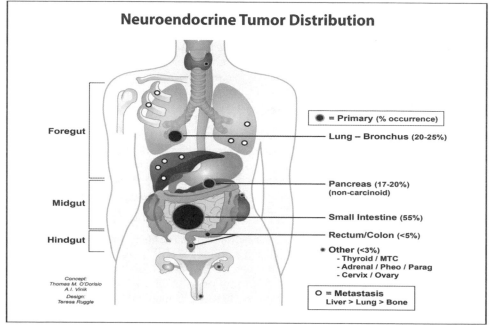

© University of Iowa

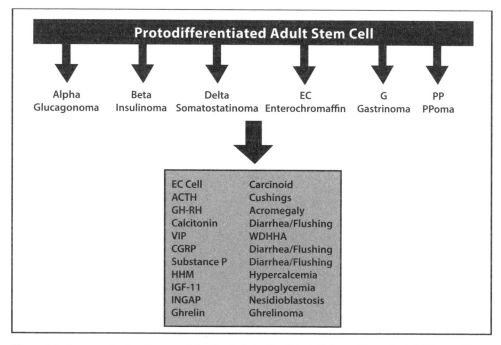

Figure 1-1. Neuroendocrine Tumors of the Gastrointestinal Tract (Adapted from Kvols LK, Perry RR, Vinik AI, et al. Neoplasms of the neuroendocrine system and neoplasms of the gastroenteropancreatic endocrine system. In: Bast RC Jr, Kufe DW, Pollock RE, et al, eds. Cancer Medicine, 6th ed. BC Dekker; 2003:1121-72.)

In some cases, multiple peptides or hormones are responsible for symptoms, and several organs and/or multiple tumors may be involved in the disease state, confounding the clinical diagnosis. To facilitate the diagnostic process, this text classifies GEP syndromes according to their secretory products and the clinical disorder they produce.

Carcinoid, gastrinoma, insulinoma, somatostatinoma, glucagonoma, and watery diarrhea (WDHHA) syndromes are described as individual syndromes according to their secretory hormones and peptides. Distinguishing signs and symptoms of each syndrome will further aid the diagnosis. These tumors can be subdivided into two main groups:
1. Orthoendocrine tumors secrete the normal product of the cell type (e.g., α-cell glucagon).
2. Paraendocrine tumors secrete a peptide or amine that is foreign to the organ or cell of origin.

Specific tumor syndromes, their clinical manifestations, and the tumor products are indicated in **(Table 1-1).**

Table 1-1. The Clinical Presentations, Syndromes, Tumor Types, Sites, and Hormones

Clinical Presentation	Syndrome	Tumor Type	Sites	Hormones
Flushing	Carcinoid	Carcinoid	Gastric, mid, and foregut, pancreas/foregut, adrenal medulla	Serotonin, NKA, SubstanceP, TCT, PP, CGRP, VIP
Diarrhea	Carcinoid	Carcinoid	As above	As above
	WDHHA	VIPoma	Pancreas, mast cells	VIP
	ZE	Gastrinoma	Pancreas, duodenum	Gastrin
	MCT	Medullary carcinoma	Thyroid, pancreas	Calcitonin
	PP	PPoma	Pancreas	PP
Diarrhea/ Steatorrhea	Somatostatin	Somatostatinoma, neurofibromatosis	Pancreas, duodenum, bleeding GI tract	Somatostatin
Wheezing	Carcinoid	Carcinoid	Gut/pancreas, lung	Serotonin, substance P, chromogranin A
Dyspepsia, Ulcer Disease, Low pH on Endoscopy	ZE	Gastrinoma Type 2 Gastric Carcinoid	Pancreas (85%), duodenum (15%) Gastric	Gastrin Gastrin
Hypoglycemia	Whipple's triad	Insulinoma	Pancreas	Insulin
		Sarcomas	Retroperitoneal	IGF/binding protein
		Hepatoma	Liver	IGF
Dermatitis	Glucagonoma Syndrome*	Glucagonoma	Pancreas	Glucagon
	Sweet's Sydnrome**	Neuroendocrine tumors	Multiple	Unknown
	Pellagra	Carcinoid	Midgut	Serotonin
Dementia	Glucagonoma Syndrome*	Glucagonoma	Pancreas	Glucagon
	Sweet's Syndrome**	Neuroendocrine tumors	Multiple	Unknown

Diabetes	Glucagonoma	Glucagonoma	Pancreas	Glucagon
	Somatostatin	Somatostatinoma	Pancreas	Somatostatin
Deep Venous Thrombosis	Somatostatin Glucagon	Somatostatinoma Glucagonoma	Pancreas Pancreas	Somatostatin Glucagon
Steatorrhea	Somatostatin	Somatostatinoma	Pancreas	Somatostatin
Cholelithiasis/ Neurofibromatosis	Somatostatin	Somatostatinoma	Pancreas	Somatostatin
Silent/Liver Metastases	PPoma Non-functional Carcinoid	PPoma Carcinoid	Pancreas Foregut, Midgut, Hindgut	Pancreatic Polypeptide (PP)
Acromegaly/ Gigantism	Acromegaly	Neuroendocrine tumors	Pancreas	GH-RH
Cushing's	Cushing's	Neuroendocrine tumors	Pancreas	ACTH/CRF
Anorexia, Nausea, Vomiting	Hypercalcemia	Neuroendocrine tumors	Pancreas	PTHRP
Constipation, Abdominal Pain		VIPoma	Pancreas	VIP
Pigmentation		Neuroendocrine tumors	Pancreas	VIP
Postgastrectomy	Dumping, syncope, tachycardia, hypoten-sion, borborygmus, explosive diarrhea, diaphoresis, mental confusion	None	Stomach/duodenum	Osmolarity, insulin, GLP

*Glucagonoma syndrome consists of necrotizing migratory erythema with bullous formation.
**Sweet's syndrome is associated with multiple types of malignancies.

These are the common neuroendocrine tumors (NETs):
- Carcinoid
- Insulinoma
- PPoma
- Gastrinoma
- VIPoma
- Glucagonoma
- Somatostatinoma
- Multiple Endocrine Neoplasia Types 1 and 2 (MEN-1 and MEN-2)
- Other rare tumors include Ghrelinoma

The great majority of these tumors are carcinoid tumors accounting for more than half those presenting each year **(Fig. 1-2)**. The incidence of carcinoid has risen in the last 10 years, particularly those found in the stomach and ileum. Insulinomas, gastrinomas, and PPomas account for 17%, 15%, and 9% respectively, whereas the rest remain around the1% mark. These tumors are nicknamed "zebras" because of their rarity, but despite their infrequent occurrence, physicians are fascinated by their complexity and the unusual nature of their presentations. For the most part, endocrinologists make their living not by diagnosing and treating one of these tumors, but rather by *excluding* conditions that masquerade as NETs. Recent data suggests that 60-80% of pNETS may not be functional or simply may not appear to be so simply because the offending hormone or peptide has not yet been identified.

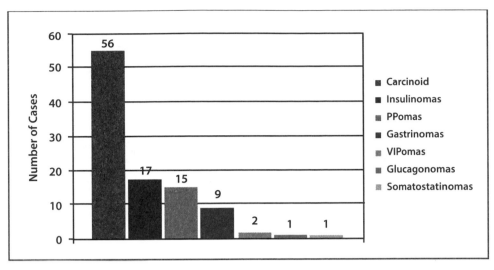

Figure 1-2. Neuroendocrine Tumors of the Gastrointestinal Tract: Annual Incidence 10 Cases per Million (From Vinik AI, Perry RR. Neoplasms of the gastroenteropancreatic endocrine system. In: Holland JF, Bast RC Jr, Morton DL, et al, eds. Cancer Medicine, vol. 1, 4th ed. Baltimore: Williams & Wilkins; 1997:1605-41.)

CHARACTERISTICS OF NEUROENDOCRINE TUMORS

- Rare
- Usually small (<1 cm)
- Slow growing (months to years, "cancer in slow motion")
- Usually metastasize to liver and bone before becoming symptomatic, often when tumor is larger than 2 cm
- Episodic expression; may be silent for years
- Often misdiagnosed; symptoms mimic commonplace conditions
- Complex diagnosis, rarely made clinically; requires sophisticated laboratory and scanning techniques

To facilitate the proper treatment regimen, diagnostic tests should be selected to:
- Determine the peptide(s) or amines responsible for the symptoms
- Locate the site and cause of the abnormality
- Eliminate other possible causes and syndromes

ICD-10 CODES for Primary Carcinoid Tumor Sites

Location	Malignant	Benign
Small intestine, unspecified portion	C7A.019	D3A.019
Duodenum	C7A.010	D3A.010
Jejunum	C7A.011	D3A.011
Ileum	C7A.012	D3A.012

Location	Malignant	Benign
Large intestine, unspecified portion	C7A.029	D3A.029
Colon NOS	C7A.029	D3A.029
Appendix	C7A.020	D3A.020
Cecum	C7A.021	D3A.021
Ascending colon	C7A.022	D3A.022
Transverse Colon	C7A.023	D3A.023
Descending colon	C7A.024	D3A.024
Sigmoid colon	C7A.025	D3A.025
Rectum	C7A.026	D3A.026

Location	Malignant	Benign
Unknown primary site, Carcinoid or Neuroendocrine NOS	C7A.00	D3A.00
Bronchus and lung	C7A.090	D3A.090
Thymus	C7A.091	D3A.091
Stomach	C7A.092	D3A.092
Kidney	C7A.093	D3A.093
Foregut NOS	C7A.094	D3A.094
Midgut NOS	C7A.095	D3A.095
Hindgut NOS	C7A.096	D3A.096
Other sites	C7A.098	D3A.098

ICD-10 CODES for Carcinoid Metastatic Sites

Secondary NET codes	
Unspecified site	C7B.00
Distant lymph nodes	C7B.01
Liver	C7B.02
Bone	C7B.03
Peritoneum	C7B.04
Other site	C7B.09

(See Carcinoid Follow-Up Profile [Chapter 5] and Flushing Syndrome Tests [Chapter 5] for specific tests and CPT codes [Chapter 4])

ICD-10 CODE: Achlorhydria K31.83

ICD-10 CODE: Carcinoid Syndrome E34.0

ICD-10 CODE: Diarrhea R19.7 NOS

ICD-10 CODE: Flushing R23.2

ICD-10 CODE: Functional Diarrhea K59.1

ICD-10 CODES for Primary NETS Sites

Sites	Malignant	Benign	Uncertain Behavior	Unspecified
Ampulla	C24.1	D13.4	D37.6	D49.0
Duodenum	C17.0	D13.2	D37.2	D49.0
Jejunum	C17.1	D13.39	D37.2	D49.0
Pancreas	C25.9	D13.6	D37.8	D49.0
Body	C25.1	D13.6	D37.8	D49.0
Head	C25.0	D13.6	D37.8	D49.0
Islet cell	C25.4	D13.7	D37.8	D49.0
Neck	C25.7	D13.6	D37.8	D49.0
Tail	C25.2	D13.6	D37.8	D49.0

(See GI–Neuroendocrine Tests [Chapter 4] for specific tests and CPT codes)

ICD-10 CODES for pNETS Metastatic Sites

Sites	Codes
Supraclavicular	C77.0
Abdominal	C77.2
Mediastinal	C77.1
Retroperitoneal	C77.2
Liver	C78.7
Bone	C79.51
Lung	C33
Brain	C71.9

ICD-10 CODES for Carcinoid Metastatic Sites

Secondary NET codes	Codes
Unspecified site	C7B.00
Distant lymph nodes	C7B.01
Liver	C7B.02
Bone	C7B.03
Peritoneum	C7B.04
Other site	C7B.09

ICD-10 CODE: Gastrinoma C25.4

ICD-10 CODE: Glucagonoma/Gastrinoma/Other Pancreatic Islet Cell Tumors
Malignant
>Pancreas C25.4 - unspecified
>Specified site–see Neoplasm by site, malignant
>Islets of Langerhans C25.4
Benign
>Pancreas D13.6–except islets of Langerhans
>Islets of Langerhans D13.7
Uncertain behavior, neoplasm of the pancreas D37.8

ICD-10 CODE: MEN-1 E31.21

ICD-10 CODE: MEN-2 E31.22

ICD-10 CODE: Sweet's Syndrome L98.2

ICD-10 CODE: Zollinger-Ellison Syndrome E16.4

ICD-10 CODES for Syndromes

Syndromes	Code
Malignant Neoplasm Pancreas, Produce Insulin, Somatostatin & Glucagon	C25.4
Islets of Langerhans	C25.4
Carcinoid Syndrome	E34.0
Zollinger-Ellison Syndrome	E16.4
Sweet's Syndrome	L98.2
MEN-I	E31.21

CARCINOID TUMORS AND THE CARCINOID SYNDROME

Carcinoid tumors are the most commonly occurring gut endocrine tumors. The prevalence of carcinoids is about 50,000 cases in any 1 year in the United States. The incidence is estimated to be approximately 1.5 cases per 100,000 of the general population (i.e., approximately 2500 new cases per year in the United States). Nonetheless, they account for 13% to 34% of all tumors of the small bowel and 17% to 46% of all malignant tumors of the small bowel. They derive from primitive stem cells known as Kulchitsky or enterochromaffin (EC) cells, originally described by Feyter as "wasser heller" or "clear water" cells and generally found in the gut wall.

Carcinoids may, however, occur in the bronchus, pancreas, rectum, ovary, lung, and elsewhere. The tumors grow slowly and often are clinically silent for many years before metastasizing. They frequently metastasize to the regional lymph nodes, liver, and, less commonly, to bone. The likelihood of metastases relates to tumor size. The incidence of metastases is less than 15% with a carcinoid tumor smaller than 1 cm but rises to 95% with tumors larger than 2 cm. In individual cases, size alone may not be the only determinant of lymphatic or distant spread. Lymphatic or vascular invasion, or spread into the fat surrounding the primary tumor, may be an indicator of a more aggressive tumor **(Table 1-2)**.

Table 1-2. Tumor Location and Frequency of Metastases (n=5468)

Gut	Location	Percentage of Tumors	Incidence of Metastases (%)
Foregut	Stomach	38	31
	Duodenum	21	33
	Lung	32.5	27
Midgut	Jejunum	2.3	70
	Ileum	17.6	70
	Appendix	7.6	35
	Colon	6.3	71
Hindgut		10	14

From Jensen RT. Carcinoid and pancreatic endocrine tumors: recent advances in molecular pathogenesis, localization, and treatment. Curr Opin Oncol.2000;12:368-77.

The carcinoid syndrome occurs in less than 10% of patients with carcinoid tumors. It is especially common in tumors of the ileum and jejunum (i.e., midgut tumors) but also occurs with bronchial, ovarian, and other carcinoids. Tumors in the rectum (i.e., hindgut tumors) rarely produce the carcinoid syndrome, even those that have widely metastasized. Tumors may be symptomatic only episodically, and their existence may go unrecognized for many years **(Fig. 1-3)**. The average time from onset of symptoms attributable to the tumor and diagnosis is just over 9 years, and diagnosis usually is made only after the carcinoid syndrome occurs. The distribution of carcinoids is Gaussian in nature. The peak incidence occurs in the sixth and seventh decades of life, but carcinoid tumors have also been reported in patients as young as 10 years of age and in those in their ninth decade. There is an overall increase in incidence of carcinoid tumors over the last decade. **(Fig. 1-4)**.

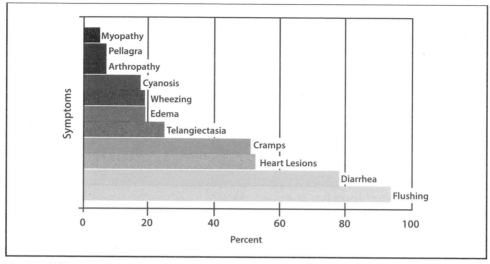

Figure 1-3. Frequency of Carcinoid Syndrome Symptoms

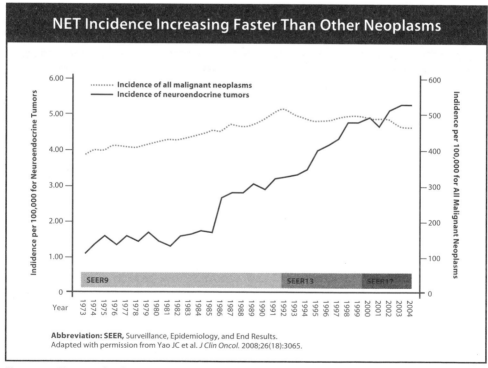

Figure 1-4. Neuroendocrine Tumors increasing faster than other neoplasms.

During the early stages, vague abdominal pain goes undiagnosed and invariably is ascribed to irritable bowel or spastic colon. At least one-third of patients with small bowel carcinoid tumors experience several years of intermittent abdominal pain before diagnosis. This pain can be due to obstruction (partial or intermittent) or to the development of intestinal angina, which in turn, may be due to bowel ischemia, especially in the postprandial period. Carcinoid tumors can present in a variety of ways. For example, duodenal tumors are known to produce gastrin and may present with the gastrinoma syndrome.

One of the more clinically useful classifications of carcinoid tumors is according to the classification of the primitive gut from which the tumor cells arise. These tumors derive from the stomach, foregut, midgut, and hindgut **(Table 1-3)**.

Table 1-3. Clinical and Biochemical Characteristics of Carcinoid Neuroendocrine Tumors

Tumor Location	Origin	Clinical Characteristics	Biochemical Characteristics
Gastric: Type 1	Secondary to achlorhydria	Pernicious anemia, atrophic gastritis, gastric polyps	gastrin <1000 pg/mL
Type 2	Hyperacidity	Larger tumors than Type 1	gastrin >1000 pg/mL
Type 3	Normal acidity	Larger tumors than Type 1 or 2, more aggressive tumor growth	Gastrin normal
Foregut		Atypical carcinoid, ZE, acromegaly, Cushing's, etc.	5-HTP
Midgut		Classic carcinoid syndrome	Serotonin, substance P, CGRP, kinins, and peptides
Hindgut		Silent	Nonsecretory

GASTRIC CARCINOID

There are three types of gastric carcinoid tumors:
1. Type 1 gastric carcinoids are associated with achlorhydria, high gastrin levels, and multiple, small, relatively nonaggressive tumors. These tumors are more common in patients with achlorhydria accompanied by pernicious anemia and vitamin B12 deficiency, in which there is loss of gastric acid secretion causing impairment of the normal restraint mechanism suppressing gastrin production. Gastrin is trophic to EC cells in the stomach, and when levels rise above 1000 pg/mL, this constitutes a threshold for the induction of gastric carcinoid polyps and tumors.
2. Type 2 gastric carcinoids are associated with elevated gastric acid, high gastrin levels, and the Zollinger-Ellison (ZE) syndrome. These tumors are larger and have a higher propensity to metastasize than type 1 carcinoids of the stomach.
3. Type 3 gastric carcinoids are much larger than types 1 and 2 and have a high propensity to metastasize. These tumors are sporadic and may be associated with normal gastrin and gastric acid levels. This type of gastric carcinoid is most likely to cause tumor-related deaths.

The clinical picture of type 1 gastric carcinoid, most commonly identified in a patient with evidence of pernicious anemia, is characterized by the following.
- Premature graying of the hair
- Associated autoimmune disorders
- Antibodies to gastric parietal cells and intrinsic factor
- Achlorhydria or hypochlorhydria
- Neutral pH instead of the normal highly acidic pH
- Serum gastrin level greater than 1000 pg/mL

CHRONIC PROTON PUMP INHIBITOR THERAPY MASQUERADES AS A GASTRIC CARCINOID OR GASTRINOMA.

- Chronic PPI therapy increases plasma Chromogranin A and Gastrin levels.
- Chronic PPI therapy induces hypochlorhydria or achlorhydria which increases gastrin secretion.
- Changes in biomarkers induced by PPI therapy can easily be confused with changes in biomarkers seen in NETS.

Proton pump inhibitors (PPIs) were introduced into clinical practice in the 1980s. While the initial use of these compounds was limited to the control of hyperacidity associated with Zollinger-Ellison syndrome (gastrinoma), their effectiveness rapidly amplified the clinical application of these compounds. The ability of PPIs to induce gastric achlorhydria is well known and the association between hypochlorhydria or achlorhydria and hypergastrinemia is also well established.[1]

Chromogranin A (CgA), a member of the granin family, has been widely touted as the best biomarker for the diagnosis and subsequent follow up of NETs.[2,3] The relative sizes of the CgA molecule and the pancreastatin fragment may provide significant increases in the sensitivity to detect small increases in neuroendocrine tumor volume.[4] Pancreastatin is a breakdown product of the large CgA molecule and the cleavage of pancreastatin from CgA is controlled by the action of prohormone convertase 1.

Recently, we and other groups have proposed that measurement of pancreastatin in patients with NETs may be more sensitive than the measurement of CgA levels. At least part of the increased sensitivity of pancreastatin vs. CgA concentrations in the diagnosis of NETs is related to differences in plasma concentration (ng/ml for CGA vs. pg/mL for Pancreastatin – a thousand-fold greater sensitivity).[4] While it is well known that chronic PPI use increases circulating gastrin and CgA levels, the effect of chronic PPI use on circulating pancreastatin levels had been relatively uninvestigated. **(See Table 1-4)**

In a recent prospective study by Raines et al patients enrolled used PPIs over long intervals (mean duration 3.1 ±2.5 years). Chronic PPI use resulted in significant increases in CgA levels in the control group vs. in the PPI user group (15.1±11 vs. 131±207ng/ml, p=0.005). Long term PPI use also resulted in significant increases in circulating gastrin levels (34.8±22.3 vs. 167.8±136.2pg/mL, p=0.001). In contrast, pancreastatin levels in non-PPI users and in chronic PPI users were almost identical (81.6±36.4 vs.89.4±43.4pg/mL, p= 0.46). Chronic PPI use is associated with significantly elevated gastrin and CgA levels; whereas, the circulating pancreastatin concentrations remain within normal limits.[5]

Table 1-4. PPIs decrease gastric acidity and alter NET biomarkers: differentiating drug effects versus NETs.

	Gastrin	Chromogranin A	Pancreastatin	Gastric pH
Chronic PPI Use	Elevated	Elevated	Normal	High
Type 1 Gastric Carcinoid	Elevated[a-c]	Elevated[a-d]	Normal/Elevated*	High[e,f]
Zollinger-Ellison	Elevated[g,h]	Elevated[g,h]	Elevated[h]	Low[h]
Type 2 Gastric Carcinoid	Elevated[a,h]	Elevated[a,h]	Elevated[h]	Low[e]
Midgut NETs	Normal	Elevated[i]	Elevated[j]	Normal

[a]Hou W and Schubert ML. Treatment of Gastric Carcinoids. Current Treatment Options in Gasterenterology. 2007; 10:123-133.
[b]Campana D, Nori F, Pezzilli R, et al. Gastric endocrine tumors type I: treatment with long-acting somatostatin analogs. Endocrine-Related Cancer. 2008;15:337-342
[c]Dakin GF, Warner RRP, Pomp A, Salky B, and Inabnet WB. Presentation, Treatment and Outcomes of Type 1 Gastric Carcinoid Tumors. J Surg Oncol. 2006;93:368-372.
[d]Peracchi M, Gebbia C, Basilico G, et al. Plasma chromogranin A in patients with autoimmune chronic atrophic gastritis, enterochromaffin-like cell lesions and gastric carcinoids. Eur J Endocrinol. 2005;152:443-448.
[e]Burkitt MD and Pritchard DM. Review article: pathogenesis and management of gastric carcinoid tumors. Aliment Phatmacol Ther. 2006; 24(9):1305-1320.
[f]Hung OY, Maithel SK, Willingham FF, Farris AB, and Kauh JS. Hypergastrinemia, Type 1 Gastric Carcinoid Tumors: Diagnosis and Management. J Clin Oncol. 2011;29(25):e713-e715.
[g]Hirschowitz BI, Worthington K, Mohnen J, and Haber M. Chromogranin A in patients with acid hypersecretion and/or hypergastrinanemia. Aliment Pharmacol Ther. 2007;26:869-878.
[h]Gibril F and Jensen RT. Zollinger-Ellison Syndrome Revisited: Diagnosis, Biologic Marker, Associated Inherited Disorders, and Acid Hypersecretion. Current Gastroenterology Reports. 2004; 6:454-463.
[i]DeHerder WW. Biochemistry of NETS. Best Practice and Research Clinical Endocrinology and Metabolism. 2007; 22:33-41.
[j]O'Dorisio TM, Krutzik SR, Woltering EA, et al. Development of a Highly Sensitive and Specific Carboxy-terminal Human Pancreastatin Assay to Monitor Neuroendocrine Tumor Behavior. Pancreas. 2010; 39(5):611-616.
*Based on 36 patients with Type 1 gastric carcinoid's seen at Ochsner Medical Center-Kenner's Neuroendocrine Tumor Clinic, 4/36 (11%) of patients had elevated pancreastatin levels. Patients with normal levels had non-metastatic disease. We suspect that patients with an elevated pancreastatin level had tumors outside of the stomach; however, this cannot be confirmed.

FOREGUT CARCINOID

Sporadic primary foregut tumors include carcinoids of the bronchus, stomach, first portion of the duodenum, pancreas, and ovaries. Midgut carcinoid tumors derive from the second portion of the duodenum, the jejunum, the ileum, and the right colon. Hindgut carcinoid tumors include those of the transverse colon, left colon, and rectum. This distinction assists in distinguishing a number of important biochemical and clinical differences among carcinoid tumors because the presentation, histochemistry, and secretory products are quite different **(see Table 1-4)**. Foregut carcinoids are argentaffin negative. They have a low content of serotonin (5-hydroxytryptamine [5-HT]). They often secrete the serotonin precursor 5-hydroxytryptophan (5-HTP), histamine, and a multitude of polypeptide hormones. Their functional manifestations include carcinoid syndrome, gastrinoma syndrome, acromegaly, Cushing's disease, and a number of other endocrine disorders. Furthermore, they are unusual in that flushing tends to be of protracted duration, is often purplish or violet instead of the usual pink or red, and frequently results in telangiectasia and hypertrophy of the skin of the face and upper neck. The face may assume a leonine appearance after repeated episodes. It is not unusual for these tumors to metastasize to bone.

MIDGUT CARCINOID

Midgut carcinoids, in contrast, are argentaffin positive, have high serotonin content, rarely secrete 5-HTP, and often produce a number of other vasoactive compounds such as kinins, prostaglandins (PGs), and substance P. The clinical picture that results is the classic carcinoid syndrome of flushing and diarrhea with or without wheezing. These tumors may produce adrenocorticotropic hormone (ACTH) on rare occasions and infrequently metastasize to bone.

HINDGUT CARCINOID

Hindgut carcinoids are argentaffin negative, rarely contain serotonin, rarely secrete 5-HTP or other peptides, and usually are silent in their presentation. However, they may metastasize to bone. A further point of interest is that a gender variation is present when a carcinoid tumor coexists with MEN-I; more than two-thirds of the time the tumor is in the thymus in males; whereas, in females, more than 75% of the time it is in the lung.

References:
1. Laine L, Ahnen D, Mcclain C, Solcia E, Walsh JH. Review article: potential gastrointestinal effects of long-term acid suppression with proton pump inhibitors. Aliment Pharmacol Ther. 2000; 14(6):651–668.
2. Woltering EA, Hilton RS, Zolfoghary CM, Thomson J, Zietz S, Go VLW, Vinik AI, Vinik E, O'Dorisio TM, Mamikunian G. Validation of serum versus plasma measurements of chromogranin A levels in patients with carcinoid tumors: lack of correlation between absolute chromogranin a levels and symptom frequency. Pancreas. 2006; 33(3):250-4.
3. Vinik AI, Silva MP, Woltering EA, Go VLW, Warner RR, Caplin M. Biochemical Testing for Neuroendocrine Tumors (NETs). Pancreas. 2009; 38(8):876-89.
4. O'Dorisio TM, Krutzik SR, Woltering EA, Lindholm E, Joseph S, Gandolfi AE, Wang Y-Z, Boudreaux JP, Vinik AI, Go VLW, Howe JR, Halfdanarson T, O'Dorisio, MS, Mamikunian G. Development of a highly sensitive and Specific carboxy-terminal Human Pancreastatin Assay to Monitor Neuroendocrine Tumor Behavior. Pancreas. 2010; 39(5):611-616.
5. Raines D, Chester M, Diebold AE, et al. A Prospective Evaluation of the Effect of Chronic Proton Pump Inhibitor Use on Plasma Biomarker Levels in Humans. Pancreas. 2012; 41:508-511.

WHAT TO LOOK FOR

Distinguishing Signs and Symptoms

The frequency of symptoms in patients with NETS include the following:
- Flushing   84 %
- Diarrhea   79%
- Hypertension   50%
- Diabetes, Metabolic Syndrome NASH   37%
- Heart Disease   37%
- Bronchoconstriction   17%
- NeuroMyopathy   7%
- Pigmentation, arthropathy   5%
- Hyper-hypoglycemia (NIHHPS)   <1%
- Ulcer disease, skin rashes   <1%
- Psychological Disturbances   <1%
- Fever, fatigue, weight loss   <1%
    - Tumor Production of Cytokines (TNF-Alpha, Interleukin 6, NFκβ)
    - Tumor Stimulation of antibody formation (Calcium Channels(P, Q), Acetylcholine receptors, cANCA, pANCA, Hu)

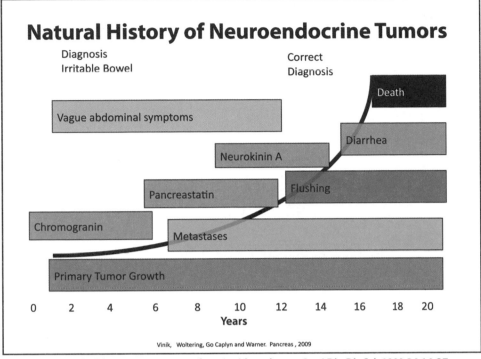

Figure 1-5. Modified from management of carcinoid syndrome. Am J Dig Dis Sci. 1989;34:14-27.

Assessment of the concurrence of the two major symptoms of carcinoid tumors reveals that flushing and diarrhea occur simultaneously in 58% of cases, diarrhea without flushing in 15%, flushing without diarrhea in 5%, and neither flushing nor diarrhea as a symptom complex in 22%. The natural history of these tumors is illustrated in **Fig. 1-5**. Invariably the patient has a long history of vague abdominal symptoms, a series of visits to his or her primary care practitioner, and referral to a gastroenterologist, often with a misdiagnosis of irritable bowel syndrome (IBS). These symptoms persist with a median latency to correct diagnosis of 9.2 years by which time the tumor has metastasized, causing flushing and diarrhea and progressing on its slow but relentless course until the patient dies. Clearly, a greater index of suspicion and a carcinoid tumor profile screen is warranted for all patients presenting with "traditional IBS symptoms." The diagnosis of metastases to the liver is generally more obvious, but often still takes place only after a delay of many years. Even then, an incorrect diagnosis is not uncommon. Unless biopsy material is examined for the secretory peptide chromogranin, synaptophysin, or neuron- specific enolase (NSE), tumors may be labeled erroneously as adenocarcinoma, with a negative impact on physicians' attitudes regarding management and underestimation of prospects for survival. **(See Fig. 1-6.)**

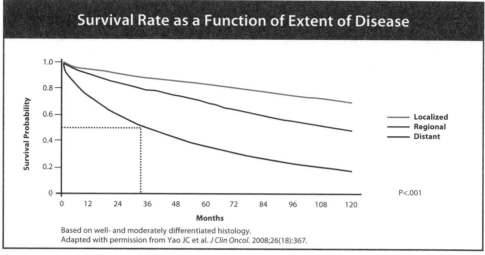

Figure 1-6. Survival rate as a function of extent of disease

NETs summary:

- GEP NETs are now the second most prevalent GI malignancy.
- Over 60% of GEP NETs are metastatic at diagnosis.
- Symptoms are often absent or vague.
- No known tests for early diagnosis.
- Survival is a function of the extent of the disease (see Figure 1-6).
- New syndromes develop that are related to NETS.

INTRODUCTION TO CHROMOGRANINS

Chromogranins belong to a unique family of secretory chromogranin and secreto-granin proteins. Chromogranin A (CgA) is an acidic protein co-released with catechol-amines during exocytosis from sympathetic nerve terminals and chromaffin cells.

Chromogranin A (CgA) determination for diagnosis and follow-up in patients with gastroenteropancreatic endocrine tumors (GEP-ET) and MEN-1is considered the standard of care in many institutions. Although the absolute value of a single measurement of CgA is not a determinate of tumor bulk nor the presence or absence of metastasis, the trend in serial CgA levels over time has been proven to be a useful predictor of tumor growth. Changes in CgA levels of more than 25% over baseline are considered significant.

Serial measurements (every 3 to 6 months) of CgA levels in blood can be used to monitor the progression of a variety of gut-derived NETs. Serum CgA level is also an effective tumor marker in patients with pheochromocytoma. Increased levels strongly correlate with tumor mass. The concordance between CgA level and the results of iodine-131 meta-iodobenzylguanidine (131I-MIBG) scintigraphy is high. A CgA level in the reference range is highly predictive of normal scintigraphy findings.

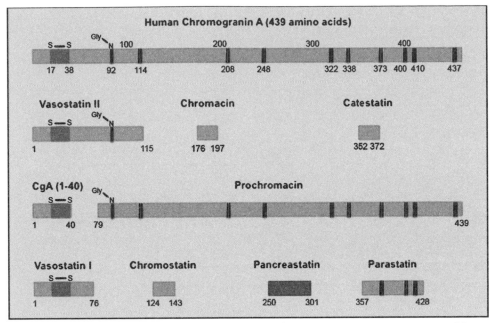

Figure 1-7. Schematic representation of CgA and its postulated biologically active sequences with the sites of proteolytic cleavage at dibasic acids indicated (vertical lines).Gly-N indicates putative N-linked glycosylation site; S-S, sites of a disulfide linkage. The numbers below each sequence refer to the location in CgA.[5]

CgA levels may also be elevated in several other endocrine and nonendocrine diseases. It is well known that drugs that suppress gastric acid secretion can increase gastrin levels. Proton-pump inhibitors (PPI) are extensively used to treat patients with ZE syndrome, gastroesophageal reflux disease (GERD) or acid–peptic disease, but their long-term use can cause significant increases in gastrin levels and cause hypertrophy of the EC cells of the stomach. Enterochromaffin-like (ECL) cell hyperplasia secondary to hypergastrinemia also leads to increased levels of CgA in blood. Treatment with inhibitors of acid secretion, atrophic gastritis, and infection with *Helicobacter pylori* are common conditions leading to hypergastrinemia. These ECL cells are the precursor cells for the development of gastric carcinoids. An increase in CgA levels quickly follows the start of low dosages of PPI. Chronic high-dose PPI use can cause persistent elevations of CgA levels for months after discontinuing PPI therapy.

Renal insufficiency and severe hypertension have been associated with increases in CgA levels. Although antihypertensive drugs do not commonly interfere with the analysis of CgA levels, some false-positive results occur in the presence of renal impairment, hypergastrinemia, corticosteroid therapy, and the use of PPI as previously mentioned. CgA has a circadian rhythm unrelated to plasma catecholamines; thus, collection of blood for serial measurement of CgA levels should be done at approximately the same time of day.

PANCREASTATIN APPEARS TO BE A MORE SENSITIVE BIOMARKER THAN CHROMOGRANIN A IN MIDGUT PATIENTS

- Pancreastatin is a fragment of the CgA molecule
- CgA is degraded to Pancreastatin by prohormone convertase PC-1
- Pancreastatin is capable of early detection of a NET
- Measurement of Pancreastatin reflects response to therapy
- Refer to above figure 1-7

Recent information suggests that CgA is a prohormone subject to intracellular and extracellular conversion to the smaller peptide, pancreastatin (49 amino acid residues).[1,2] Prohormone convertase-1 (PC-1) seems to be an important endoprotease that is responsible for this conversion.[3] In addition to pancreastatin's multiple intermediary metabolic actions in vivo, recent articles suggest that, like CgA, pancreastatin may have value as both a NETs biomarker and possibly as a prognostic indicator of malignant tumor behavior.

The pancreastatin assays published to date use antibodies that cross-react in varying percentages with the larger prohormone, CgA. This makes it difficult to accurately interpret the impact that PC-1 may have in the various stages of malignant NETs. Furthermore, larger tumor burden may be needed to detect changes in CgA that are measured in quantities of nanograms per milliliter (ng/mL). Thus, it is possible that the measurement of pancreastatin may better reflect both the maturity of a NET and, perhaps, be a sensitive and specific marker of early increases in tumor activity/burden. Pancreastatin is measured in picograms per milliliter (pg/mL), rather than nanograms per milliliter and, thus, is 1,000-fold more sensitive than CgA.

O'Dorisio et al. recently reported the development of a pancreastatin radioimmunoassay (RIA) that is highly specific and sensitive (pg/mL) for the active carboxy-terminal region of human pancreastatin 1-52 with negligible CgA crossreactivity. Their goal was to demonstrate the utility of pancreastatin as a marker of liver tumor progression and report parallelism of split patient samples of pancreastatin between our novel new assay and a previously published pancreastatin assay that measures both CgA and pancreastatin. They also attempted to demonstrate the utility of serial pancreastatin measurements as a sensitive marker of liver tumor progression in patients with metastatic NETs and to demonstrate its sensitivity in a series of patients undergoing extensive cytoreductive surgery.

Further support of the sensitivity of pancreastatin as a measure for the effectiveness of therapeutic intervention can be made from an ongoing study of hepatic cytoreduction procedures in patients with metastatic NETs from Louisiana State University in New Orleans. Thirty-nine patients with metastatic carcinoid tumor of the small intestine and elevated preoperative pancreastatin and CgA levels underwent greater than 90% hepatic cytoreduction. Determination of the percent of tumor cytoreduced was made independently by two surgeons who estimated tumor burden after reduction. Of the 39 patients with elevated preoperative pancreastatin levels, 38 (97%) exhibited greater than 25% decrease in pancreastatin after 90% hepatic cytoreduction. The overall mean ± SD pancreastatin decrease in the debulked population was 53% ± 44%.. In contrast to the 39 patients with elevated preoperative CgA levels, only 17 (44%) exhibited greater than 25% CgA decreases after 90% hepatic cytoreductive surgery. Clearly, pancreastatin was a much more sensitive biomarker with respect to the percent tumor debulked during cytoreductive surgery than was CgA.

Whether greater than 25% decrease in pancreastatin levels after major liver tumor cytoreduction predicts stabilization of tumor burden, as was previously reported, remains to be determined. In light of the work of Desai et al., Calhoun et al., the recent work of Bloomston et al., and our group's collaborative efforts, we conclude that C-terminally directed pancreastatin assays may provide us with an important early marker of changes in NET burden, especially metastatic disease in the liver.[4] This concept was recently alluded to by Stronge et al. from Belfast, UK. Using antibodies raised in rabbits to synthetic human pancreastatin and specific to the C-terminal region of pancreastatin (as in the present assay in the United States), these authors demonstrated that an immediate increase in pancreastatin after initiation of somatostatin analog therapy was associated with poor patient survival.

References:
1. Woltering EA, Hilton RS, Zolfoghary CM, Thomson J, Zietz S, Go VLW, Vinik AI, Vinik E, O'Dorisio TM, Mamikunian G. Validation of serum versus plasma measurements of chromogranin A levels in patients with carcinoid tumors: lack of correlation between absolute chromogranin a levels and symptom frequency. Pancreas. 2006; 33(3):250-4.
2. O'Dorisio TM, Krutzik SR, Woltering EA, Lindholm E, Joseph S, Gandolfi AE, Wang Y-Z, Boudreaux JP, Vinik AI, Go VLW, Howe JR, Halfdanarson T, O'Dorisio MS, Mamikunian G. Development of a highly sensitive and Specific carboxy-terminal Human Pancreastatin Assay to Monitor Neuroendocrine Tumor Behavior. Pancreas. 2010; 39(5):611-616.
3. Endocrinology & Metabolism Clinics of North America. Vinik AI ed. Ardill JE, O'Dorisio TM, Vol. 1, page 777-790, 2010.
4. Ito T, Igarashi H, Jensen RT. Serum Pancreastatin: the long sought universal, specific tumor marker for neuroendocrine tumors? Pancreas. 2012;41:505-507.

THE NEXT STEP

Diagnosis

The diagnosis of carcinoid tumors rests on a strong clinical suspicion in patients who present with flushing, diarrhea, wheezing, myopathy, and right-sided heart disease and includes appropriate biochemical confirmation and tumor localization studies.

Biochemical Studies

The rate-limiting step in carcinoid tumors for the synthesis of serotonin is the conversion of tryptophan into 5-HTP, catalyzed by the enzyme tryptophan hydroxylase. In midgut tumors, 5-HTP is rapidly converted to serotonin by the enzyme aromatic amino acid decarboxylase (dopa-decarboxylase). Serotonin is either stored in the neurosecretory granules or may be secreted directly into the vascular compartment. Most of the secreted serotonin is taken up by platelets and stored in their secretory granules. The rest remains free in the plasma, and circulating serotonin is then converted into the metabolite 5-hydroxyindoleacetic acid (5-HIAA) by the enzymes monoamine oxidase and aldehyde dehydrogenase. These enzymes are abundant in the kidney, and the urine typically contains large amounts of 5-HIAA.

In patients with foregut tumors, the urine contains relatively little 5-HIAA but large amounts of 5-HTP. It is presumed that these tumors are deficient in dopa-decarboxylase; this deficiency impairs the conversion of 5-HTP into serotonin, leading to 5-HTP secretions into the vascular compartment. Some 5-HTP, however, is converted to serotonin and 5-HIAA, producing modest increases in levels of these metabolites.

5-HIAA: PLASMA VERSUS URINE

The normal range for a 24 hour urinary collection of 5-HIAA varies between laboratories, but is approximately 6-8 mg per day and the quantitation of serotonin and all of its metabolites usually permits the detection of 84% of patients with carcinoid tumors. No single measurement detects all cases of carcinoid syndrome, although the urine 5-HIAA appears to be a commonly used screening procedure. Other peptides involved include substance P, neuropeptide K, pancreatic polypeptide (PP), pancreastatin, neurokinin A, neuropeptide Y, and CgA.

Given the potential problems and inconveniences for patients associated with collecting a 24-hour urine sample, including adhering to strict dietary requirements, ISI set out to develop a practical and accurate plasma 5-HIAA assay that would provide results that were equivalent to the urinary 5-HIAA. The ISI plasma 5-HIAA assay was tested in a limited number of subjects with a variety of tumors. Other groups have attempted to measure 5-HIAA from plasma, and have found it to be a reliable method that gives results comparable to urinary 5-HIAA.

The most common 24 hour urinary 5-HIAA collection protocol involves discarding the first morning urine on the collection day and then collecting all urine in a chilled container over the next 24 hour period. The first urine on the following morning is considered part of the collection and is also deposited into the container. Collection and refrigeration of the 24 hour urine specimen is extremely inconvenient, especially if it requires collecting urine at the workplace. Different testing facilities vary in their requirements as far as what type of collection jug to use and what type of preservatives (if any) need to be in the jug. If these requirements are not followed exactly, the collection often has to be repeated. When queried most patients tell you that they spend about half of a day getting the proper collection jug, one day collecting the specimen and then another half day returning the collection container to the laboratory. While this time expenditure does not directly affect the cost of the urinary 5-HIAA assay, it certainly needs to be considered as part of the overall cost and usefulness of the biomarker determination.

Based on the potential for diet to affect the concentration of serotonin in the blood most physicians suggest that for 48 hours prior to the collection of urinary 5-HIAA, patients should abstain from red wine, avocado, walnuts, cheese, hot dogs, chocolates, vanilla-containing foods, custard, pineapple, kiwi, bananas, and cassava. However, the plasma 5-HIAA assay by ISI shows clearance rates for serotonin are less than 8 hours. Therefore, the only requirement for the plasma 5HIAA assay is an overnight fast. Drugs can also alter 5-HIAA urine values, such as acetanilide, phenacetin, glyceryl guaiacolate (found in many cough syrups), methocarbamol, and reserpine. Drugs that can decrease urinary 5-HIAA levels include heparin, isoniazid, levodopa, monoamine oxidase inhibitors, methenamine, methyldopa, phenothiazines, and tricyclic antidepressants.[1]

The ISI plasma 5-HIAA assay alleviates these issues and only requires collection with ISI's Z-tube™ preservative following a simple overnight fast (8 hours). See collection instructions in Chapter 4.
- **Plasma 5-HIAA and urinary 5-HIAA levels correlate closely implying that a fasting plasma 5-HIAA can be used instead of 24-hour urinary 5-HIAA.**
- Plasma 5-HIAA and urinary 5-HIAA provide similar clinical information in midgut NETs patients.
- Plasma 5-HIAA collection is much more convenient than a 24-hour urine collection.

References:
1. Tellez MR, Mamikunian G, O'Dorisio TM et al. A single fasting plasma 5-HIAA value correlates with 24-hour urinary 5-HIAA values and other biomarkers in midgut neuroendocrine tumors (NETs). Pancreas. 2013:42(3): 405-410.
2. Hande KR. Multiple-organ syndromes: Carcinoid syndrome. In: Goldman L, Ausiello D, eds. Cecil Medicine. 23rd ed. Philadelphia, PA: Saunders Elsevier; 2007: Ch 251.

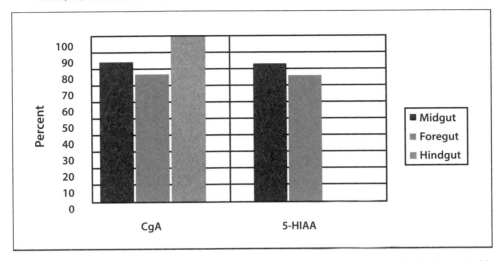

Figure 1-8. Chromogranin A Versus 5-HIAA urine in Neuroendocrine Tumors (From Vinik AI. Carcinoid tumors. In: DeGroot LJ, Jameson JL, eds. Endocrinology, vol. 3, 4th ed. Philadelphia, PA: WB Saunders; 2001:2533-58.) Note the lack of 5-HIAA levels in hindgut tumors.

Figure 1-8 shows the percent positivity of CgA versus urinary 5-HIAA in the different carcinoids. CgA is positive 80% to 100% of the time in fore-, mid-, and hindgut tumors; whereas, 5-HIAA detects a little more than 70% of midgut tumors, reveals only 30% of foregut tumors, and fails to recognize the presence of a hindgut carcinoid tumor. Evaluating PP levels in conjunction with CgA levels may further enhance this sensitivity. Both markers were measured in 68 patients (28 functioning and 40 nonfunctioning tumors). CgA sensitivity was 96% in functioning tumors and 75% in nonfunctioning tumors, and 74% in pancreatic and 91% in gastrointestinal tumors. Specificity was 89%.

Biomarkers in NETs

In contrast to CgA alone, pancreastatin sensitivity for NETs was approximately 50%, but combining the two markers increased sensitivity for all tumors to greater than 95%. More specifically, the gain in detection of pancreatic tumors was 93% with CgA and pancreastatin versus 68% using CgA alone. It seems reasonable to recommend using both markers under these circumstances. There are, however, always caveats. Gastric parietal cell antibodies neutralize acid secretion thereby unbridling the G-cell to produce gastrin that is trophic to the gastric ECL cells. Following a period of progressive hypertrophy, these ECL cells can transform into gastric carcinoid. Measurement of gastrin and CgA, but not NSE and 5-HIAA, is a means of evaluating the ECL mass. This is particularly useful in therapeutic decision-making with regard to doing an antrectomy or simply following conservatively and removing carcinoid polyps as they arise. Of course, this raises the issue of whether reported elevations in CgA in people taking PPI are truly false-positive or reflect ECL hyperplasia. Recent evidence from Rainers et al demonstrated that PPI's do not affect circulating pancreastatin levels. This makes pancreastatin a valuable tool to rule out the PPI effect on other biomarkers. Evidence points to the combined measurement of the following biomarkers:

- 5-HIAA (Plasma or urine)
- CgA
- Pancreastatin
- Gastrin
- Gastric pH
- Antiparietal cell antibody

These measurements are a very effective means of discovering a NET, identifying its probable site of origin, and monitoring response to intervention. In carcinoid tumors, neurotensin is elevated in 43% of patients, substance P in 32%, motilin in 14%, somatostatin in 5%, and vasoactive intestinal polypeptide (VIP) rarely.

Common amines and peptides produced by carcinoids that cause symptoms are as follows:
- Serotonin
- Histamine
- Substance P

The following constitute the best clinical practice panel of markers for diagnosis and follow-up of carcinoid tumors:
- CgA
- 5-HIAA (Plasma or urine)
- Gastrin
- Serotonin
- Pancreastatin
- Neurokinin A (NKA; substance K)

In patients who are not responding to octreotide or lanreotide clinically or biochemically or in those who exhibit tumor progression, measurement of the octreotide/ lanreotide level will help determine appropriateness of drug dosing. Quantification of plasma hormonal responses to octreotide suppression may help in the prediction of long-term responses to therapy.

NEUROKININ A (NKA) AS A PREDICTOR OF SURVIVAL IN PATIENTS WITH MIDGUT NETs

- NKA levels less than 50 pg/mL predict a greater than 90% 2-year survival in midgut NETS patients.
- Persistently elevated NKA levels greater than 50 pg/mL predict poor 2-year survival (approximately 50%).
- NKA values that exceed 50 pg/mL but fall to levels that are less than 50 pg/mL following therapy also have a greater than 90% 2-year survival re rates.

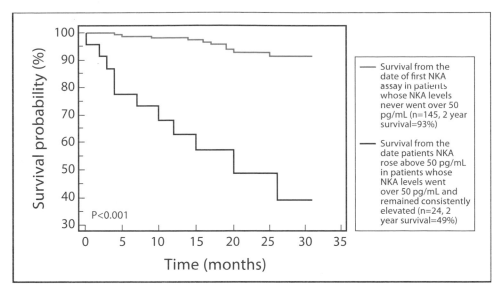

Figure 1-9. This Kaplan-Meier survival curve shows the overall survival of patients with persistently normal (<50 pg/mL) NKA values vs. the survival of individuals whose NKA was persistently >50 pg/mL. The difference in median survival of these two groups was highly statistically significant (p<.0001).[1]

Serial determination of neurokinin A (NKA) levels may be extremely useful for the identification of midgut neuroendocrine tumor patients with a poor prognosis. Turner et al. demonstrated that NKA is a useful independent marker of prognosis and that low (< 50 pg/mL) circulating NKA plasma levels are strongly associated with enhanced survival. These authors believe that NKA can also aid in the early identification of patients with more aggressive tumors, allowing for better clinical management of these patients. Ardill et al. demonstrated that survival and NKA levels are inversely proportional. In her study, patients with NKA levels persistently over 50 pg/mL (ng/L) had a three year survival rate of 10%. Conversely, patients with NKA levels consistently less than 50 pg/mL had a three year survival rate of 65%. Patients with NKA levels that rose above 50 pg/mL, but then subsequently returned to less than 50 pg/mL following therapy had the same survival as those patients that never had an elevated NKA value.

Recently, Woltering et al. cross-validated the results of the European NKA assay (Royal Infirmary, Belfast Northern Ireland) with a commercial NKA assay offered in the United States by ISI (Inter Science Institute - Inglewood CA).[1] In the validation study, plasma samples were sent from the United States to Northern Ireland and additional plasma samples were sent from Northern Ireland to the United States. The Northern Ireland NKA assay uses an extraction step before assay, while the United States assay does not. In spite of the technical differences in these two assays, the results of both assays were essentially identical. Based on this study, and the studies by Ardill's group, we hypothesized that patients from the United States with well differentiated midgut NETS whose serial NKA values are consistently below 50 pg/mL will have an excellent short term prognosis compared to the short term survival of patients with NKA values that remain consistently greater than 50 pg/mL before and after the introduction of somatostatin.[2] Survival after the introduction of somatostatin is also better than the pre-somastatin era. **(See Fig. 1-9)**

Reference:
1. Mamikunian P, Ardill JE, O'Dorisio TM, Krutzik SR, Vinik AI, Go VLW, Armstrong L, Mamikunian G, Woltering EA. Validation of Neurokinin A assays in the United States and Europe.Pancreas 2011;40:1000-1005.
2. Diebold AE, Boudreaux JP, Wang YZ, Anthony LB, Uhlhorn AP, Ryan P, Mamikunian P, Mamikunian G, and Woltering EA. Neurokinin A levels predict survival in patients with well differentiated small bowel neuroendocrine tumors. Surgery. Accepted.

ICD-10 CODE: Carcinoid Syndrome E34.0

ICD-10 CODES for Carcinoid Primary Tumor Sites

Location	Malignant	Benign
Small intestine, unspecified portion	C7A.019	D3A.019
Duodenum	C7A.010	D3A.010
Jejunum	C7A.011	D3A.011
Ileum	C7A.012	D3A.012

Location	Malignant	Benign
Large intestine, unspecified portion	C7A.029	D3A.029
Colon NOS	C7A.029	D3A.029
Appendix	C7A.020	D3A.020
Cecum	C7A.021	D3A.021
Ascending colon	C7A.022	D3A.022
Transverse colon	C7A.023	D3A.023
Descending colon	C7A.024	D3A.024
Sigmoid colon	C7A.025	D3A.025
Rectum	C7A.026	D3A.026

Location	Malignant	Benign
Unknown primary site, Carcinoid or Neuroendocrine NOS	C7A.00	D3A.00
Bronchus and lung	C7A.090	D3A.090
Thymus	C7A.091	D3A.091
Stomach	C7A.092	D3A.092
Kidney	C7A.093	D3A.093
Foregut NOS	C7A.094	D3A.094
Midgut NOS	C7A.095	D3A.095
Hindgut NOS	C7A.096	D3A.096
Other sites	C7A.098	D3A.098

ICD-10 CODES for Carcinoid Metastatic Sites: Secondary Neuroendocrine

Secondary NET codes	
Unspecified site	C7B.00
Distant lymph nodes	C7B.01
Liver	C7B.02
Bone	C7B.03
Peritoneum	C7B.04
Other site	C7B.09

(See Carcinoid Follow-Up Profile [Chapter 5] and Flushing Syndrome Tests [Chapter 5] for specific tests and CPT codes [Chapter 4])

GASTRINOMA (ZOLLINGER-ELLISON SYNDROME)

Gastrinoma (Zollinger-Ellison syndrome-ZES) is characterized by hyperacidity and gastrin hypersecretion from an islet cell tumor (gastrinoma) of the pancreas or duodenum. Approximately 90% of gastrinomas are found in the "gastrinoma" triangle, an area bordered by the confluence of the cystic and common ducts superiorly, the mesenteric vessels medially, and the lateral sweep of the "C" loop of the duodenum laterally. A primary gastrinoma is rarely found in the liver or ovary, and even more rarely in a lymph node. These tumors may be associated with peptic perforation, obstruction, hemorrhage, and/or hyperacidity. Atrophic gastritis, pernicious anemia, gastric carcinoid, chronic proton pump inhibitor use, and diabetic gastropathy may produce spuriously high gastrin levels. A high gastrin level in the absence of diarrhea suggests atrophic gastritis. Gastric pH measurement remains a valuable tool in distinguishing the causes of hypergastrinemia. Even though this measurement is easily performed, it is often overlooked.

WHAT TO LOOK FOR

Distinguishing Signs and Symptoms

- Mean age of patients with sporadic gastrinomas is 48–55 years; 54–56% are males.
- Mean delay in diagnosis from the onset of symptoms is 5.2 years. All of the symptoms except those late in the disease course are due to gastric acid hypersecretion.
- The majority of ZES patients present with a single duodenal ulcer or
- Gastroesophageal Reflux Disease (GERD) symptoms and ulcer complications.
- Multiple ulcers or ulcers in unusual locations are a less frequently presenting feature than in the past.
- Abdominal pain primarily due to PUD or GERD occurs in 75–98% of the cases, Diarrhea in 30–73%, heartburn in 44–56%, bleeding in 44–75%, nausea/vomiting in 12–30% weight loss in 7–53%.
- At presentation, 98% of patients have an elevated fasting serum gastrin level,
- 87–90% have marked gastric acid hypersecretion (basal acid output greater than 15 mEq/h) and 100% have a gastric acid pH < 2.
- Patients with Multiple Endocrine Neoplasia Type 1 (MEN-1) with ZES (20–30%) present at an earlier age (mean 32–35 years) than patients without MEN-1 (i.e. sporadic disease). In 45% of MEN-1/ZES patients, the symptoms of ZES precede those of hyperparathyroidism, and can be the initial symptoms these patients present with.
- However, almost all MEN-1/ ZES patients have hyperparathyroidism at the time the ZES is diagnosed, although in many patients it can be asymptomatic and mild and therefore can be easily missed if ionized calcium and serum parathormone levels are not performed.
- Twenty-five percent of all MEN-1/ZES patients lack a family history of MEN-1, supporting the need to screen all ZES patients for MEN-1.

THE NEXT STEP

Gastrinoma (ZES) should be suspected if: recurrent, severe or familial PUD is present; PUD without H. pylori is present; PUD resistant to treatment or associated with complications (perforation, penetration, bleeding) is present; PUD occurs with endocrinopathies or diarrhea; PUD occurs with prominent gastric folds on barium studies or at endoscopy (present –92% of ZES patients), or with hypercalcemia or hypergastrinemia.

Biochemistry/Laboratory Studies for Gastrinoma (ZES)

Diagnosis of gastrinoma syndrome depends on the demonstration of:
- elevated serum gastrin levels
- a positive secretin stimulation test
- gastric acid hypersecretion

Initially to make the diagnosis, fasting serum gastrin (FSG) and gastric pH should be determined (following interruption of PPI for at least 1 week with H2-blocker coverage, if possible). If FSG is 10-fold elevated and gastric pH < 2, then a secretin test and basal acid output should be performed. Also, if repeated fasting serum gastrin tests are performed on different days, 0.5% of ZES patients will have all normal values.

Elevated Serum Gastrin Level

Normal values of gastrin are 100 to 120 pg/mL. Proton Pump Inhibitor (PPI) will raise levels to 400 to 500 pg/mL, and can also occasionally be higher. Fasting gastrin concentrations greater than 500 pg/mL in the presence of normal or excess gastric acid is suspicious of gastrinoma. Very high levels of greater than 1000 pg/mL may be pathognomonic of gastrinoma. Pernicious anemia and atrophic gastritis can produce gastrin levels greater than 1000 pg/mL, which should alert the clinician to the possibility of gastric carcinoid. Hypergastrinemia in the absence of increased acid production is not due to gastrinoma. Recent data suggests that if using antacids or PPI's, a pancreastatin test should also be ordered at the same time as gastrin to differentiate from tumor-related gastrin.[1]

Serum gastrin levels are usually greater than150 pg/mL in patients with gastrinoma syndrome. The exception is a small fraction of patients who secrete a biologically active variant not recognized by the antiserum used for the assay. A careful history and physical is required, as gastrin levels may be elevated for a variety of other reasons (**Table 1-5**). Measurement of gastric pH is also useful, because in the absence of antisecretory drugs, a pH of 3.0 or higher excludes Zollinger-Ellison Syndrome.

Table 1-5. Causes of Hypergastrinemia

With increased acid	With decreased acid
Gastrinoma	Atrophic gastritis
G-cell hyperfunction	Pernicious anemia
Gastric outlet obstruction	Vagotomy
Short bowel syndrome	Gastric carcinoma
Retained antrum	Renal disease
Hypercalcemia	Rheumatoid arthritis
Hyperparathyroidism	Vitiligo
MEN-1	Diabetic pseudo ZE syndrome; PPI sue
MEN-1 = Multiple endocrine neoplasia type 1; ZE = Zollinger-Ellison	

Positive Secretin Stimulation Test

The most accurate and sensitive test for the diagnosis of Gastrinoma remains the secretin stimulation test for gastrin secretion. No new test has emerged with a greater sensitivity or specificity. Secretin, 2 U/kg is given intravenously, and blood samples for gastrin are drawn at baseline 2, 5,10, 20, and 30 minutes. A rise of more than 100 pg/mL is strongly suggestive of Zollinger-Ellison Syndrome (ZES). False positive results are rare, and are usually found in hypochlorhydric states. G-cell (gastrin cell) hyperplasia syndrome can be sometimes confused with the gastrinoma syndrome. Patients with G-cell hyperplasia typically have an equivocal response to secretin stimulation, and an exaggerated response to food ingestion, thus distinguishing them from patients with gastrinoma.

Gastric Acid Hypersecretion

Establishment of the presence of gastric acid hypersecretion should include measurements of volume as well as basal and pentagastrin-stimulated acid secretion. The diagnosis is confirmed if: a) the volume of gastric secretion is large, typically greater than 10 liters per 24 hours; b) the basal acid output is over 15 mmol/h. Values in the 10-15 range are borderline, and less than 10 mmol/h exclude diagnosis of Zollinger-Ellison Syndrome. In patients who have previously undergone vagotomy, basal acid output in gastrinoma is over 3 mmol/h; c) the ratio of basal acid output to maximal pentagastrin stimulated acid output is greater than 0.6.

MEN-1 should be suspected if there is a family or personal history of endocrinopathies or recurrent peptic disease; history of renal colic or nephrolithiases; history of hypercalcemia or pancreatic endocrine tumor syndromes.

References
1. Raines D, Chester M, Diebold AE, Mamikunian P, Anthony CT, Mamikunian GM, Woltering EA. A Prospective evaluation of the effect of chronic proton pump inhibitor use on plasma biomarker levels in humans. *Pancreas* 2012;41:508-511.
2. Ito T, Igarashi H, Jensen RT. The long sought universal, sensitive, specific tumor marker for neuroendocrine tumors? *Pancreas* 2012;41:505-507.

Biochemistry/Laboratory Studies for MEN-1/ZES

All patients with Gastrinoma (ZES) should have serum parathormone levels (preferably an intact molecule assay – IRMA), fasting calcium levels and prolactin levels measured. Recent studies show that an ionized calcium level is much more sensitive than a total calcium- or albumin corrected-calcium determination.

Genetic Study for MEN-1

- If the family history is positive for MEN-1, suspicious clinical or laboratory data for MEN-1 are found or multiple tumors are present raising the possibility of MEN-1, then MEN-1 genetic testing should be done. If the genetic testing is positive for MEN-1, genetic counseling should be performed.
- Ectopic Cushing's syndrome develops in 5–15% of patients with advanced metastatic disease and has a very poor prognosis.
- It should be routinely assessed for in patients with advanced metastatic disease by careful clinical examination, history and routine 24-hour urinary cortisol determinations and serum cortisol and ACTH assessment. Elevation of calcitonin also carries a poorer prognosis.
- A secondary hormonal syndrome develops in 1–10% of patients, especially those with metastatic disease or MEN-1. These should be assessed for by a careful clinical history and routine hormonal assays are not recommended.
- Test for MEN-1 gene.

Tumor localization studies are required in all patients with Gastrinoma (ZES) biochemically established.

Most recommend initially a UGI endoscopy with careful inspection of the duodenum followed by a helical CT and Somatostatin Receptor Scintigraphy (SRS) (Octreoscan, Mallinckrodt Medical. St. Louis, Missouri). If these studies are negative and surgery is being considered, endoscopic ultrasound should be performed. If results are still negative, selective angiography with secretin stimulation and hepatic venous sampling should be considered. SRS is the best study to initially stage the disease and detect both liver and distant metastases. Intraoperative ultrasound and routine duodenotomy for duodenal lesions preferably preceded by transillumination of the duodenum should be done in all patients at surgery. Bone metastases occur in up to one-third of patients with liver metastases and should be sought in all patients by using SRS and an MRI of the spine. Measurement of bone alkaline phosphatase and N Telopeptide may be useful markers of bone involvement. **(See Table 1-6)**

Table 1-6. Methods of Tumor Localization in Gastrinoma

Tests Percentage	Ultrasound	Infusional CT	Computed tomography	SRS	Selective angiography	Secretin angiography	THVS PTHVS Local	PTHVS Regional
Sensitivity	21	40	31	71	60, 29	89	35	94
Specificity	92	100	66	86	100, 100	100	89	97
Positive predictive value	80	100	83	85	100, 100	---	---	94
Negative predictive value	44	50	15	52	60,100	---	89	---

PTHVS = percutaneous transhepatic portal, pancreatic, and hepatic venous gastrin sampling. Data from Norton and colleagues, Jensen, as well as Vinik and colleagues.

ICD-10 CODE: Dyspepsia K30

ICD-10 CODE: Peptic Ulcer
Without obstruction K27.9
With obstruction K27.9
With hemorrhage-
Without obstruction K27.4
With obstruction K27.4
And perforation-
Without obstruction K27.6
With obstruction K27.6

ICD-10 CODE: Zollinger-Ellison/Gastrinoma E16.4
Malignant
Carcinoid of duodenum C7A.010
Islet of Langerhans C25.4
Gastric Carcinoid Type II I C7A.092
Pancreatic islet cell neoplasm C25.4
Stomach C7A.092
Specified site-see Neoplasm by site, malignant
Unspecified site C25.9
Benign
Abnormality of gastrin secretion E16.4
Duodenum D13.2
Pancreatic islet cell neoplasm D13.7
Stomach D3A.092
Unspecified site D37.9
Uncertain behavior, see Neoplasm
Gastric Carcinoid Type II C7A.092

(See Table 1-1 for primary tumor sites and common metastatic tumor site) (See Gastrin Test [Chapter 4] for specific requirements and CPT codes. See Secretin Stimulation test requirements [Chapter 6].)

References
1. Wang JS, Boudreaux JP, Anthony LB, Campeau R, Raines D, O'Dorisio TM, Go VLW, Vinik AI, Cundiff J, Woltering EA. NETS: current recommendations for diagnosis and surgical management. Endocrinol Metab Clin North Am. 2011 Mar;40(1):205-231,x.Review.
2. Jensen RT and Gibril F. Somatostatin receptor scintigraphy in gastrinomas. Ital J Gastroenterol Hepatol.1999;31(Suppl2):179-85.
3. Vinik AI, Achem-Karam S, and Owyang C. Gastrointestinal hormones in clinical medicine. In Special Topics in Endocrinology and Metabolism.Vol. 4. eds M.P., Foa PP. New York, NY: Alan R. Liss; 1982:93-138.
4. Vinik AI, Delbridge L, Moattari R, Cho K, and Thompson N, Transhepatic portal vein catheterization for localization of insulinomas: a ten-year experience. Surgery.1991;109:1-11.
5. Norton JA, Doppman JL, Collen MJ, Harmon JW, Maton PN, Gardner JD, Jensen RT. Prospective study of gastrinoma localization and resection in patients with Zollinger-Ellison syndrome. Ann Surg.1986;204:468.
6. Vinik AI, Strodel WM, Lloyd RV, and Thompson NW. Unusual gastroenteropancreatic tumors and their hormones. Endocrine Surgery Update, eds Thompson N and Vinik AI. New York, NY: Grune & Stratton; 1983:293.

GHRELINOMA

Since its recent discovery, there have been about 650 publications on this peptide, indicating a profound interest in the newest GEP hormone capable of stimulating growth hormone (GH) release by activation of the GH secretogogue type 1a (GHS-R1a) receptor. Ghrelin is the first natural hormone in which a hydroxyl group on one of its serine residues is acylated by n-octanoic acid. This acylation is essential for binding to the GHS-R1a receptor, for the GH-releasing capacity, and also likely for its other actions. Although it has been found to co-segregate with glucagon and insulin by some authors, this is not consistent, and most would agree that its cell of origin in the pancreas constitutes a new cell type.

Ghrelin stimulates the following:
- GH release in animals and humans by acting at both the pituitary and hypothalamic level
- Release of ACTH and prolactin, gastric acid secretion, and intestinal motility
- Gastric motility and gastric acid secretion

Ghrelin regulates the following:
- Energy balance
- Increased appetite and food intake
- Modulation of insulin secretion negatively
- Exertion of a tonic inhibitory role on insulin secretion in animals and humans
- Suppressed by hyperglycemia and insulin, and may, in addition, have a direct role on glycogenolysis

Ghrelin increases the following:
- Blood glucose levels
- Insulin resistance when administered systemically in humans

The expression of ghrelin protein and/or mRNA has recently been identified in almost all gastric and intestinal carcinoids as well as pancreatic NETs. There have been two case reports of ghrelinomas: in one, ghrelin was co-secreted with glucagon in a predominantly glucagon expression syndrome, whereas in the other nonfunctioning tumor, ghrelin levels were greater than 12,000 pM (normal, 300 pM).
- Current data implies that the most common association with increased Ghrelin levels is gastroparesis.
- Gastric bypass is associated with increased ghrelin levels and gastric banding is not.
- An increase in ghrelin levels may occur depending upon the assay being used and what is measured, that is acylated versus non-acylated ghrelin.

Based on the physiologic effects of ghrelin, one would expect that the clinical features of a ghrelinoma would include the following:
- Hyperglycemia
- Insulin deficiency
- Insulin resistance
- GH excess
- Increased IGF-1 levels
- Acromegaly
- Gastric acid hypersecretion
- Intestinal dysmotility

Reference:
1. Richardson DW, Mason ME, Vinik AI. In: Endocrinology & Metabolism Clinics of North America. 2010:81-96.

WHAT TO LOOK FOR

Distinguishing Signs and Symptoms

Ghrelin is a 28–amino acid acylated peptide related to the oxyntomodulin family of intestinal peptides. This peptide was isolated from the X/A-like neuroendocrine cells of the rat and human stomach. It is predominantly produced by the stomach but is also detectable in many other tissues:

- Bowel
- Hypothalamus
- Pituitary
- Pancreas
- Co-segregating with pancreatic alpha cells
- Possibly with pancreatic beta cells

Hormones and Peptides

- Ghrelin
- IGF-1
- CgA

Diagnosis

It seems for now that ghrelin is another hormone produced in some GEP NETs that has little, if any, biologic activity. Its utility as a marker for response to therapy needs more investigation. In terms of screening, ghrelin does not seem to offer a great deal over conventional markers. However, in time it may demonstrate an ability to predict tumors. The initial excitement regarding ghrelin may run a parallel course with the excitement related to the discovery of PP; like PP, ghrelin has since been found to be a nonspecific marker because of its lack of a biologic effect. The difference is that ghrelin has been shown to have many effects when administered in the acylated form, and the increase in the endogenous levels of ghrelin in these tumors may be a variant of the acylated form without biologic activity. This peptide may, however, retain sufficient structural epitopes to be recognized by the antisera to ghrelin. Acylation-specific antisera will help to resolve part of this question.

ICD-10 CODE: Acromegaly E22.0

ICD-10 CODE: Carcinoid Syndrome E34.0

ICD-10 CODE: Diarrhea NOS R19.7

ICD-10 CODE: Diabetes Type I (Insulin Deficiency)
Not stated as uncontrolled E10.9
Uncontrolled E10.65

ICD-10 CODE: Dysmetabolic Syndrome X (Insulin Resistance) E88.81

ICD-10 CODE: Gastric Acid Hypersecretion K30

ICD-10 CODE: Hyperglycemia NOS R73.9

ICD-10 CODES for Primary pNETS Tumor Sites

Sites	Malignant	Benign	Uncertain Behavior	Unspecified
Ampulla	C24.1	D13.4/D13.5	D37.6	D40.0
Duodenum	C17.0	D13.2	D37.2	D49.0
Jejunum	C17.1	D13.2	D37.2	D49.0
Pancreas	C25.9	D13.6	D37.8	D49.0
Body	C25.1	D13.6	D37.8	D49.0
Head	C25.0	D13.6	D37.8	D49.0
Islet cell	C25.4	D13.7	D37.8	D49.0
Neck	C25.7	D13.6	D37.8	D49.0
Tail	C25.2	D13.6	D37.8	D49.0

ICD-10 CODES for pNETS Metastatic Sites and Syndromes

Sites	Malignant
Supraclavicular	C77.0
Abdominal	C77.2
Mediastinal	C77.1
Retroperitoneal	C77.2
Liver	C78.7
Bone	C79.51
Lung	C33
Brain	C71.9

Syndromes	Code
Malignant Neoplasm Pancreas, Produce Insulin, Somatostatin & Glucagon	C25.4
Islets of Langerhans	C25.4
Zollinger-Ellison Syndrome	E16.4
Whipple's Syndrome	K90.81
Sweet's Syndrome	L98.2
MEN-I	E31.21

(See Oral Glucose Tolerance Test for Diabetes, Insulinoma, Impaired Glucose Tolerance, Metabolic Syndrome, PCOS, Reactive Hypoglycemia, and Acromegaly [Chapter 6], MEN Syndrome Screen [Chapter 5], and GI–Neuroendocrine Tests for specific tests and CPT codes [Chapter 4])

GLUCAGONOMA SYNDROME

In 1966, McGavran and colleagues called attention to a syndrome that included acquired diabetes and glucagon-producing tumors. Because these tumors usually were accompanied by a very characteristic skin rash, the syndrome is also known as the 4D syndrome, which stands for dermatosis, diarrhea, deep venous thrombosis (DVT), and depression.

WHAT TO LOOK FOR

Distinguishing Signs and Symptoms

- Characteristic rash (necrolytic migratory erythema [NME]) (82%)
- Painful glossitis
- Angular stomatitis
- Normochromic normocytic anemia (61%)
- Weight loss (90%)
- Mild diabetes mellitus (80%)
- Hypoaminoacidemia
- DVT (50%)
- Depression (50%)

In a study of 1366 consecutive adult autopsies, a tumor frequency of 0.8% was found. All tumors were adenomas, and all contained histochemically defined glucagon cells. None of the tumors had been suspected during life. Although these adenomas contained glucagon, it is not known whether they were overproducing or even secreting glucagon. The incidence in vivo is probably 1% of all NETs.

Features of the Necrolytic Migratory Erythematous Rash

The NME rash of the glucagonoma syndrome has a characteristic distribution. It usually is widespread, but major sites of involvement are the perioral and perigenital regions along with the fingers, legs, and feet. It may also occur in areas of cutaneous trauma. The basic process in the skin seems to be one of superficial epidermal necrosis, fragile blister formation, crusting, and healing with hyperpigmentation. Skin biopsy specimens usually show small bullae containing acantholytic epidermal cells as well as neutrophils and lymphocytes. The adjacent epidermis usually is intact, and the dermis contains a lymphocytic perivascular infiltrate. Different stages of the cutaneous lesions may be present simultaneously. Biopsy examination of a fresh skin lesion may be the most valuable aid in suggesting the diagnosis of glucagonoma syndrome, but repeated biopsy samples may be necessary to confirm the diagnosis. A painful glossitis manifested by an erythematous, mildly atrophic tongue has been associated with the cutaneous lesions.

Two other features of the syndrome are noteworthy:
1. A high rate of thromboembolic complications, particularly pulmonary embolism and the unexplained occurrence of arterial thrombosis. Unexplained thromboembolic disease should alert one to the possibility of glucagonoma. (In some studies, anticoagulation therapy with warfarin has been ineffective). Most authors recommend heparin-based therapy for patients with this complication of glucagonoma.
2. Depression and other psychiatric disturbances.

Other metabolic disorders associated with cutaneous lesions may closely resemble the NME of the glucagonoma syndrome. These include:
- Acrodermatitis enteropathica
- Zinc deficiency induced by hyperalimentation
- Essential fatty acid deficiency
- Dermatosis of protein calorie malnutrition of kwashiorkor
- Pellagra resulting from niacin deficiency

Cutaneous manifestations associated with malabsorptive states often are nonspecific, affecting approximately 20% of patients with steatorrhea.

Glucose Intolerance

Glucose intolerance in the glucagonoma syndrome may relate to tumor size. Fasting plasma glucagon levels tend to be higher in patients with large hepatic metastases than in those without hepatic metastases, and all patients with large hepatic metastases have glucose intolerance. Massive hepatic metastases may decrease the ability of the liver to metabolize splanchnic glucagon, thus increasing peripheral plasma glucagon levels. Glucagon may not directly induce hyperglycemia, however, unless metabolism of glucose by the liver is directly compromised.

THE NEXT STEP

Measure plasma glucagon concentrations by radioimmunoassay. In patients with glucagonomas, fasting plasma glucagon concentrations may be as high as 2100 ± 334 pg/mL. These levels are markedly higher than those reported in normal, fasting subjects (i.e., <150 pg/mL) or in those with other disorders causing hyperglucagonemia, including diabetes mellitus, burn injury, acute trauma, bacteremia, cirrhosis, renal failure, or Cushing's syndrome, in which fasting plasma glucagon concentrations often are elevated but remain less than 500 pg/mL.

Hormones and Peptides

As with other islet cell neoplasms, glucagonomas may overproduce multiple hormones:
- Glucagon
- Insulin
- CgA
- PP
- Parathyroid hormone (PTH)
- Substances with PTH-like activity
- Gastrin
- Serotonin
- VIP and Alpha or Beta and Gamma-melanocyte-stimulating hormone (MSH), in that order of frequency

Measure the following:
- Plasma glucagon
- Insulin
- ACTH, PP
- Gastrin
- Serotonin
- VIP
- PTH
- Parathyroid hormone–related peptide (PTHRP)

Reference
1. McGavran MH, Unger RH, Recant L, Polk HC, Kilo C, Levin ME. A glucagon-secreting α-cell carcinoma of the pancreas. N Engl J Med. 1966 June 23;274(25):1408-13.

ICD-10 CODE: Glucagonoma C25.4

Malignant
    Islet cell neoplasm C25.4
    Unspecified site C25.9
    Specified site–see Neoplasm by site, malignant
Benign
    Pancreas D13.7
    Unspecified site D13.7
Uncertain behavior, neoplasm of the pancreas D37.8
Islet cell neoplasm D13.7

ICD-10 CODES for Primary pNETS Tumor Sites

Sites	Malignant	Benign	Uncertain Behavior	Unspecified
Ampulla	C24.1	D13.4/D13.5	D37.6	D40.0
Duodenum	C17.0	D13.2	D37.2	D49.0
Jejunum	C17.1	D13.2	D37.2	D49.0
Pancreas	C25.9	D13.6	D37.8	D49.0
Body	C25.1	D13.6	D37.8	D49.0
Head	C25.0	D13.6	D37.8	D49.0
Islet cell	C25.4	D13.7	D37.8	D49.0
Neck	C25.7	D13.6	D37.8	D49.0
Tail	C25.2	D13.6	D37.8	D49.0

ICD-10 CODES for pNETS Metastatic Sites and Syndromes

Sites	Malignant
Supraclavicular	C77.0
Abdominal	C77.2
Mediastinal	C77.1
Retroperitoneal	C77.2
Liver	C78.7
Bone	C79.51
Lung	C33
Brain	C71.9

Syndromes	Code
Malignant Neoplasm Pancreas, Produce Insulin, Somatostatin & Glucagon	C25.4
Islets of Langerhans	C25.4
Zollinger-Ellison Syndrome	E16.4
Sweet's Syndrome	L98.2
MEN-I	E31.21

(See GI-Neuroendocrine Tests for specific tests and CPT codes [Chapter 4])

INSULINOMAS

The classic description of insulinoma is of Whipple's triad, which includes symptoms of hypoglycemia with a low blood glucose concentration relieved by the ingestion of glucose. These tumors are most commonly benign (90%) and can be located anywhere within the pancreas. Insulinomas are associated with a memory rule known as "the rule of tens," which refers to the following characteristics: 10% are malignant; 10% are ectopic; and 10% are related to the MEN-1syndrome. Removal of the tumor, which is invariably in the pancreas, is curative in more than 90% of cases.

Adult-onset nesidioblastosis is a rare condition in which islets become hypertrophied and produce excess insulin. The diagnostic differentiation of an insulinoma from adult-onset nesidioblastosis is possible only by histologic evaluation of sufficient pancreatic tissue; fine needle biopsy does not obtain a specimen of adequate quantity. In the newborn, hypoglycemia and excess insulin production can be caused by nesidioblastosis; insulinomas are rare in this age group.

WHAT TO LOOK FOR

Distinguishing Signs and Symptoms

The major symptoms of an insulinomas are those of hypoglycemia, which can be adrenergic:
- Nervousness
- Sweating
- Palpitations
- Diaphoresis (profuse sweating)
- Circumoral tingling

Central nervous system symptoms include the following:
- Blurred vision
- Confusion
- Disorientation
- Memory loss leading to coma
- Stupor
- If chronic, dementia

THE NEXT STEP

The blood glucose level alone is not diagnostic for insulinoma, nor in general is the absolute insulin level elevated in all cases of organic hyperinsulinism (see Hypoglycemia in Chapter 2). The standard diagnostic test remains a 72-hour fast while the patient is closely observed. More than 95% of cases can be diagnosed based on their response to this test. Serial glucose and insulin levels are obtained every 4 hours over the 72-hour period until the patient becomes symptomatic. When symptoms occur, obtain insulin, glucose, and C-peptide levels. Because the absolute insulin level is not elevated in all patients with insulinomas, a normal level does not rule out the disease; however, a fasting insulin level of greater than 24 µU/mL is found in approximately 50% of patients with insulinoma. This is strong evidence in favor of the diagnosis. Values of insulin greater than 7 µU/mL after a more prolonged fast in the presence of a blood glucose level less than 40 mg/dL are also highly suggestive. A refinement in the interpretation of glucose and insulin levels has been established by determining the ratio of insulin levels in microunits per milliliter to the concomitant glucose level in milligrams per deciliter. An insulin/glucose ratio greater than 0.3 has been found in virtually all patients proven to have an insulinoma or other islet cell disease causing organic hyperinsulinism. Calculating the amended insulin/glucose ratio as follows can increase the accuracy of the test:

amended ratio = insulin (μU/mL)/glucose (mg/dL) − 30 normal <50

If the amended ratio is greater than 50, then organic hyperinsulinism is certain. Measurements of proinsulin and C-peptide have proven to be valuable in patients suspected of having organic hypoglycemia. Normally, the circulating proinsulin concentration accounts for less than 22% of the insulin immunoreactivity but is greater than 24% in more than 90% of individuals with insulinomas. Furthermore, a proinsulin level greater than 40% is highly suspicious for a malignant islet cell tumor. The C-peptide level is useful in ruling out fictitious hypoglycemia from self-administration of insulin. Commercial insulin preparations contain no C-peptide, and combined with high insulin levels, low C-peptide levels confirm the diagnosis of self-administration of insulin. High-performance liquid chromatography to characterize the insulin species found in the blood was useful before the advent of recombinant human insulin, which is not distinguishable from native insulin. Patients who take sulfonylureas surreptitiously may have increased insulin and C-peptide values soon after ingestion, but chronic use will result in hypoglycemia without increased insulin or C-peptide levels. Only an index of suspicion and measurement of urine sulfonylureas will lead to the correct diagnosis. A variety of insulin stimulation and suppression tests were used before precise and accurate insulin measurements were available. Each had its limitations, and all are currently considered obsolete. The insulin response to secretin stimulation (2 U/kg intravenously; peak response in 1–5 minutes) is a valuable measure to differentiate multiple adenomas from nesidioblastosis and single adenomas. The normal maximal increase is 74 μU/mL, whereas in single adenomas it is only 17 μU/mL, in nesidioblastosis it is 10 μU/mL, and in two patients with multiple B-cell adenomas and hyperplasia, the increases were 214 and 497 μU/mL. Patients with single adenomas and nesidioblastosis do not respond to secretin, whereas those with multiple adenomas or hyperplasia have an excessive insulin response to the administration of secretin.

Hormones and Peptides

- Insulin
- Proinsulin
- C-peptide

The standard diagnostic test is a 72-hour fast while the patient is closely observed. More than 95% of cases can be diagnosed based on responses to a 72-hour fast (see 72-Hour Supervised Fast for the Diagnosis of Insulinoma, Chapter 6). Symptomatic hypoglycemia must be accompanied by a correspondingly low blood glucose value (<50 mg/dL) with relief of symptoms by the administration of glucose.

ICD-10 CODE: Insulinomas C25.4
Malignant
Unspecified site C25.4
Specified site–see Neoplasm by site, malignant
Islet cell neoplasm C25.4
Benign, unspecified site D13.6
Islet cell neoplasm C25.4
Uncertain behavior, neoplasm of pancreas D37.8
Islet cell neoplasm C25.4

ICD-10 CODES for pNETS Sites

Sites	Malignant	Benign	Uncertain Behavior	Unspecified
Ampulla	C24.1	D13.4/D13.5	D37.6	D40.0
Duodenum	C17.0	D13.2	D37.2	D49.0
Jejunum	C17.1	D13.2	D37.2	D49.0
Pancreas	C25.9	D13.6	D37.8	D49.0
Body	C25.1	D13.6	D37.8	D49.0
Head	C25.0	D13.6	D37.8	D49.0
Islet cell	C25.4	D13.7	D37.8	D49.0
Neck	C25.7	D13.6	D37.8	D49.0
Tail	C25.2	D13.6	D37.8	D49.0

ICD-10 CODES for pNETS Metastatic Sites and Syndromes

Sites	Malignant
Supraclavicular	C77.0
Abdominal	C77.2
Mediastinal	C77.1
Retroperitoneal	C77.2
Liver	C78.7
Bone	C79.51
Lung	C33
Brain	C71.9

Syndromes	Code
Malignant Neoplasm Pancreas, Produce Insulin, Somatostatin & Glucagon	C25.4
Islets of Langerhans	C25.4
Carcinoid Syndrome	E34.0
Zollinger-Ellison Syndrome	E16.4
Sweet's Syndrome	L98.2
MEN-I	E31.21

(See 72-Hour Supervised Fast for the Diagnosis of Insulinoma [Chapter 6], Oral Glucose Tolerance Test for Diabetes, Insulinoma, Impaired Glucose Tolerance, Metabolic Syndrome, PCOS, Reactive Hypoglycemia, and Acromegaly [Chapter 6], and Hypoglycemia/Insulinoma Screening Test [Chapter 6] for specific tests and CPT codes [Chapter 4])

MULTIPLE ENDOCRINE NEOPLASIA SYNDROMES (MEN)

MEN 1

- Pituitary gland
- Pancreas
- Parathyroid glands

The pituitary tumors are primarily prolactinomas, the pancreatic tumors are PPomas, and the gastrinomas, with rare instances of insulinoma, are more commonly nesidioblastosis or hyperplasia of beta cells and parathyroid hyperplasia rather than adenoma. These tumors are associated with the loss of a tumor suppressor gene on chromosome 11q13. This is the same chromosome on which the insulin gene has been located. It has been suggested, but not proven, that allelic losses in the MEN-1 tumor suppressor gene located in the 11q13 region also might be responsible for sporadic parathyroid and pituitary tumors as well as NETs of the stomach, pancreas, and intestine. The few cases of carcinoid tumors studied have not shown losses in the 11q13 region.

MEN 2a

Multiple endocrine neoplasia type 2a (MEN-2a) syndrome is characterized by the occurrence of the following tumors:
- Pheochromocytomas
- Medullary carcinoma of the thyroid (MCT)
- Parathyroid hyperplasia

MEN 2b

Multiple endocrine neoplasia type 2b (MEN-2b), has stigmata of cutaneous and mucosal neuromas and is not associated with parathyroid hyperplasia. MEN-2a and MEN-2b and familial MCT are associated with mutations of the RET protooncogene, which is a conventional dominant oncogene located on 10q11.2. Although mutations in this region have been associated with sporadic MCT, the role, if any, of this gene in sporadic GEP tumors is not known. Occasionally there are crossover syndromes in which features of one syndrome occur in the milieu of the other syndrome (e.g., pheochromocytomas appearing in MEN-1).

Diagnosis

Diagnostic tests for the following:
- MCT
- Calcitonin
- Calcium infusion
- RET protooncogene
- Pheochromocytoma
- Vanillyl mandelic acid (VMA), epinephrine, norepinephrine
- Glucagon stimulation
- ^{131}I-MIBG

Clinical Suspicion

- Hypertension, sustained or paroxysmal (90% - 40/50)
- Headache

- Excessive truncal sweating
- Palpitations
- Pallor more common than flushing
- Anxiety/nervousness/panic
- Early on (familial or incidental adrenal mass – up to 49% in recent series) normotensive/asymptomatic – 10%

Unusual Presentations

- Dyspnea
- Nausea, anorexia
- Weight loss
- Weakness
- Visual disturbances
- Acute psychosis
- Diabetes

Very Unusual Presentations

- Myocardial infarction
- Pulmonary edema
- Arrhythmias
- Dilated Cardiomyopathy
- Autonomic dysfunction
  - Orthostatic hypotension
  - Acute bladder outlet obstruction
  - Constipation
  - Erectile dysfunction

ICD-10 CODE: MEN-1 E31.21

ICD-10 CODE: MEN-2A E31.22

ICD-10 CODE: MEN-2B E31.23

ICD-10 CODES for Endocrine Cell Tumor Sites

Site	Malignant	Benign	Uncertain Behavior	Unspecified
Pancreas	C25.9	D13.6	D37.8	D49.0
Body	C25.1	D13.6	D37.8	D49.0
Head	C25.0	D13.6	D37.8	D49.0
Islet cell	C25.4	D13.7	D37.8	D49.0
Neck	C25.7	D13.6	D37.8	D49.0
Tail	C25.2	D13.6	D37.8	D49.0
Pituitary gland	C75.1	D35.2	D44.3	D49.7
Parathyroid gland	C75.0	D35.1	D44.2	D49.7
Thyroid	C73	D34	D44.0	D49.7
Adrenal	C74.9	D35.00	D44.10	D49.0

ICD-10 CODES for pNETS Metastatic Sites and Syndromes

Sites	Malignant
Supraclavicular	C77.0
Abdominal	C77.2
Mediastinal	C77.1
Retroperitoneal	C77.2
Liver	C78.7
Bone	C79.51
Lung	C33
Brain	C71.9

Syndromes	Code
Malignant Neoplasm Pancreas, Produce Insulin, Somatostatin & Glucagon	C25.4
Islets of Langerhans	C25.4
Carcinoid Syndrome	E34.0
Zollinger-Ellison Syndrome	E16.4
Sweet's Syndrome	L98.2
MEN-1	E31.21

(See MEN Syndrome Screen [Chapter 5] for specific tests and CPT codes [Chapter 4])

PHEOCHROMOCYTOMA

The classic triad of symptoms and signs of Pheochromocytoma are headache palpitations and sweating. This symptom complex has a high specificity (93.8%) and sensitivity (90.9%) for the diagnosis of Pheochromocytoma[6], but it may be completely asymptomatic[7] and thus frequently go undiagnosed[7,8]. The frequency of these symptoms in patients with proven pheochromocytomas is not all that high. Palpitations occur in (50%), tachycardia (40%), sweating (30%) and headaches (20%). Hypertension may be labile, but patients may be normotensive or rarely hypotensive particularly if the tumor secretes only epinephrine. Complications of pheochromocytoma are mostly due to the oversecretion of norepinephrine and include sudden death, heart failure due to toxic cardiopathy, hypertensive encephalopathy, cerebrovascular accidents or neurogenic pulmonary edema[3,9]. Weight loss is usual (one never sees a fat pheochromocytoma); heat intolerance and insulin resistance with hyperglycemia are metabolic features of Pheochromocytoma patients.

Pheochromocytomas may be discovered incidentally during a surgical procedure, during investigations for the symptom complex and even after diagnosis of an adrenal incidentaloma.

When to suspect pheochromocytoma

- Hyperadrenergic cells, such as
  - Self-limited episodes of nonexertional palpitations, diaphoresis, headache, tremor or pallor
- Resistant hypertension
- A familial syndrome that predisposes to catecholamine-secreting tumors, such as
  - MEN 2, NF1, VHL
- A familial history of pheochromocytoma
- An incidentally discovered adrenal mass
- Hypertension and diabetes
- Pressor response during anesthesia, surgery or angiography
- Onset of hypertension at a young age (less than 20 years)
- Idiopathic dilated cardiomyopathy
- A history of gastric stromal tumor or pulmonary chondromas (Carney triad)

Differential diagnosis of Pheochromocytoma

The differential diagnosis of Pheochromocytoma is: hyperthyroidism, hypoglycemia, mastocytosis, carcinoid syndrome, menopause, heart failure, arrhythmias, migraine, epilepsy, porphyria, lead poisoning, panic attacks, and fictitious disorders, such as the use of cocaine and benzedrine.

Diagnostic tests for Pheochromocytoma

If the diagnosis of Pheochromocytoma is suspected, measure catecholamines or their metabolites in plasma or urine. Unfortunately, many conditions increase circulating epinephrine and Norepinephrine i.e.: stress or hypothyroidism or exogenous intake of sympathomimetic drugs. In contrast, some pheochromocytomas secrete intermittently and the circulating levels or urine levels of catecholamines may be entirely normal. On the contrary, metabolites of epinephrine and norepinephrine, metanephrines and normetanephrine are produced almost exclusively by Pheochromocytoma tissues (93-94%) and are at a constant rate independent of their release from storage vessicles[10]

making them the most sensitive and specific measures for pheochromocytoma.
(See Table 1-7) One has to be certain to exclude certain medications: methyldopa;
sympathomimetic, such as amphetamines; vasodilators, such as nitrates or
hydrallazine; alpha adrenergic antagonists, such as phenoxybenzamine and prazosin;
beta blockers, tricyclics and antidepressants. Cigarette smoking, marijuana and
cocaine use can also interfere with the assay. Alcohol, clonidine withdrawal, essential
hypertension and anxiety can produce erroneous results.

Table 1-7. Sensitivity and specificity for test with Pheochromcytoma

Tests	Sensitivity %	Specificity %
Plasma catecholamines	84	81
Plasma free total metanephrines	100	97
Urine total Metanephrines	77	93
Vanillylmandelic acid (VMA)	64	95
Urine catecholamines	86	88

Plasma free metanephrines are the most sensitive tests for screening and diagnosis of
pheochromocytoma[11]. The combined assay of plasma free metanephrines has 100%
sensitivity and 96.7% specificity and a negative predictive value of 100%[3,6, 10]. A negative
test rules out pheochromocytoma with high probability. Clonidine suppression tests
are now rarely used because of the induction of hypotension and stimulation with
glucagon may be hazardous due to increase in hypertensive crisis.

Tumor Characteristics

- Approximately 95% of catecholamine secreting tumors are in the abdomen:
- 85 – 90 percent of which are intraadrenal (pheochromocytoma)
- 5 to 10 percent of these are multiple
- Approximately 10-15% of catecholamine secreting tumors are extra-adrenal and
  are referred to as catecholamine-secreting paraganglianomas.

Malignant potential

It is difficult to predict the development of malignancy of a pheochromocytoma
based upon the site of the tumor or the histology thereof unlike the situation in
carcinoid. Furthermore these tumors may be multicentric so that only the primary
tumors in sites in which there is no chromaffin tissue can be considered to have
metastasis. The most common sites are the bones, lungs, liver and lymph nodes. In
general tumors > 5cm and extra-adrenal tumors are likely to metastasize. The size of
the tumor is an unreliable predictor of malignancy in that site[14]. Hereditary factors
should also be considered and confirmed with genetic testing. **(See Table 1-8)**

- About 10 percent of all catecholamine-secreting tumors are malignant (8.5 % in
  one report and 13% in another)
- Malignant pheochromocytomas are histologically and biochemically the
  same as benign ones. The only reliable clue to the presence of a malignant
  pheochromocytoma is local invasion or distant metastases, which may occur as
  long as 20 years after resection.
- A quick way to remember is using the rule of 10's:
  10% are malignant, 10% are extra-adrenal and 10% are bilateral

Table 1-8. Hereditary Forms of Pheochromocytoma

Syndrome	Gene	Gene Location	Frequency of Pheochromocytoma
MEN II	RET oncogene	10q11	30-50%
VH-L	Von Hippel Landau suppressor gene	3p25	15-20%
Neurofibromatosis Type 1	Neurofibromatosis Type 1	17q11	1-5%
Familial Carotid Body Tumors	Paraganlioma	11q21-23	

References:
1. Cryer PE: Pheochromocytoma. West J Med. 1992;156:399-407.
2. Scholz T, Eisenhofer G, Pacak K, Dralle H, Lehnert H: Clinical review: Current treatment of malignant pheochromocytoma. J Clin Endocrinol Metab 2007;92:1217-1225.
3. Lenders JW, Eisenhofer G, Mannelli M, Pacak K: Phaeochromocytoma. Lancet. 2005;366:665-675.
4. Yadav S, Singh SK, Sharma SK, Puri PK: Extra-adrenal pheochromocytoma: a cause of ureteral obstruction. J Urol. 2000;163:264.
5. Lenders JW, Pacak K, Eisenhofer G: New advances in the biochemical diagnosis of pheochromocytoma: moving beyond catecholamines. Ann N Y Acad Sci. 2002;970:29-40.
6. Westphal SA: Diagnosis of a pheochromocytoma. Am J Med Sci. 2005;329:18-21.
7. Mitchell L, Bellis F: Phaeochromocytoma–"the great mimic": an unusual presentation. Emerg Med J. 2007;24:672-673.
8. Cohen DL, Fraker D, Townsend RR: Lack of symptoms in patients with histologic evidence of pheochromocytoma: a diagnostic challenge. Ann N Y Acad Sci. 2006;1073:47-51.
9. Lin PC, Hsu JT, Chung CM, Chang ST: Pheochromocytoma underlying hypertension, stroke, and dilated cardiomyopathy. Tex Heart Inst J. 2007;34:244-246.
10. Vaclavik J, Stejskal D, Lacnak B, Lazarova M, Jedelsky L, Kadalova L, Janosova M, Frysak Z, Vlcek P: Free plasma metanephrines as a screening test for pheochromocytoma in low-risk patients. J Hypertens. 2007;25:1427-1431.
11. Garg A, Banitt PF: Pheochromocytoma and myocardial infarction. South Med J. 2004;97:981-984.
12. Cohen DL, Fraker D, Townsend RR: Lack of symptoms in patients with histologic evidence of pheochromocytoma: a diagnostic challenge. Ann N Y Acad Sci. 2006;1073:47-51.
13. Dimas S, Roukounakis N, Kafetzis I, Bethanis S, Anthi S, Michas S, Kyriakou V, Kostas H: Feasibility of laparoscopic adrenalectomy for large pheochromocytomas. JSLS. 2007;11:30-33.
14. Brogsitter C, Pinkert J, Bredow J, et al. Enhanced tumor uptake in neuroendocrine tumors after intraarterial application of 131I-MIBG. J Nucl Med 46. 2005;(12):2112-2116.

ICD-10 CODE: Malignant Neoplasm of the Thyroid Gland C73

ICD-10 CODE: Hyperparathyroidism E21.3
ICD-10 CODE: Pheochromocytoma
Malignant
    Specified site–see Neoplasm by site, malignant
    Unspecified site C74.10
Benign
    Specified site–see Neoplasm by site, benign
    Unspecified site D35.00
Uncertain behavior
    Adrenal neoplasm D44.10
    Neoplasm of bladder D49.4
    Neoplasm of sympathetic nervous system D43.9

ICD-10 CODE: Polyglandular Activity in MEN-I E31.21
ICD-10 CODE: Polyglandular Activity in MEN-IIA E31.22
ICD-10 CODE: Polyglandular Activity in MEN-IIB E31.23

ICD-10 CODES for Endocrine Cell Tumor Sites

Site	Malignant	Benign	Uncertain Behavior	Unspecified
Pancreas	C25.9	D13.6	D37.8	D49.0
Body	C25.1	D13.6	D37.8	D49.0
Head	C25.0	D13.6	D37.8	D49.0
Islet cell	C25.4	D13.7	D37.8	D49.0
Neck	C25.7	D13.6	D37.8	D49.0
Tail	C25.2	D13.6	D37.8	D49.0
Pituitary gland	C75.1	D35.2	D44.3	D49.7
Parathyroid gland	C75.0	D35.1	D44.2	D49.7
Thyroid	C73	D34	D44.0	D49.7
Adrenal	C74.9	D35.00	D44.10	D49.0

ICD-10 CODES for pNETS and Syndromes

Sites	Malignant
Supraclavicular	C77.0
Abdominal	C77.2
Mediastinal	C77.1
Retroperitoneal	C77.2
Liver	C78.7
Bone	C79.51
Lung	C33
Brain	C71.9

Syndromes	Code
Malignant Neoplasm Pancreas, Produce Insulin, Somatostatin & Glucagon	C25.4
Islets of Langerhans	C25.4
Carcinoid Syndrome	E34.0
Zollinger-Ellison Syndrome	E16.4
Sweet's Syndrome	L98.2
MEN-1	E31.21

(See MEN Syndrome Screen [Chapter 5] for specific tests and CPT codes)

PPOMA

Pancreatic polypeptide (PPoma) was discovered in 1972 by Chance and colleagues. These authors discovered and purified a single protein peak from a crude insulin preparation. In mammals, 93% of the cells producing PP are located in the pancreas. Meal ingestion, cerebral stimulation, and hormone administration have dramatic effects on circulating levels of PP. A biologic role for PP has not been established, however.

WHAT TO LOOK FOR

Distinguishing Signs and Symptoms

The only physiologic effects of PP that are recognized in humans are the inhibition of gallbladder contraction and pancreatic enzyme secretion. Thus, a tumor deriving from PP cells is expected to be clinically silent, although this is not always the case. For example, a tumor that invaded the bile ducts producing biliary obstruction was found to be a PPoma. It has been suggested that WDHHA, which is seen in GEP endocrine tumors, may have its origin in PP overproduction. The picture is complicated by the fact that mixed tumors, PP-cell hyperplasia in association with other functioning islet cell tumors, ductal hyperplasia of PP cells, nesidioblastosis, and multiple islet tumors producing PP also have been described, either alone or as part of the MEN-1 syndrome **(Table 1-9)**.

Table 1-9. Coincident Elevations of Pancreatic Polypeptide

Tumor Type	Proportion of Patients With Coincident Elevations	Pancreatic Polypeptide Level in Plasma (pg/mL) or Other Laboratory Abnormalities
Endocrine-secreting tumors	22%-77%	>1000
Carcinoid tumors	29%-50%	>1000
Adenocarcinomas	53 patients	Not elevated
Nonfunctional GEP tumors	50%-75%	Slightly raised
Nonfunctional GEP tumors	50%-75%	Secretin more elevated

A response of greater than 5000 pg/min/mL (i.e., integrated response) is more than two standard deviations (SD) above that observed in healthy persons. In the absence of factors, such as chronic renal failure, that is known to cause marked elevation of PP levels, a markedly elevated PP level in an older, healthy patient occasionally may indicate a nonfunctioning pancreatic endocrine tumor. Differentiation of a high basal concentration in a healthy person from that appearing in patients with tumor is difficult. It has been suggested that administration of atropine would suppress PP concentrations in healthy subjects and would fail to do so in patients with tumors, but this has not been subjected to extensive examination.

Reference
1. Gepts W, de Mey J. [Pancreatic polypeptide.] [Article in French.] Diabetes Metab. 1978 Dec;4(4):275-83.

ICD-10 CODES for Primary pNETS Tumor Sites

Sites	Malignant	Benign	Uncertain Behavior	Unspecified
Ampulla	C24.1	D13.4/D13.5	D37.6	D40.0
Duodenum	C17.0	D13.2	D37.2	D49.0
Jejunum	C17.1	D13.2	D37.2	D49.0
Pancreas	C25.9	D13.6	D37.8	D49.0
Body	C25.1	D13.6	D37.8	D49.0
Head	C25.0	D13.6	D37.8	D49.0
Islet cell	C25.4	D13.7	D37.8	D49.0
Neck	C25.7	D13.6	D37.8	D49.0
Tail	C25.2	D13.6	D37.8	D49.0

ICD-10 CODES for pNETS Metastatic Sites and Syndromes

Sites	Malignant
Supraclavicular	C77.0
Abdominal	C77.2
Mediastinal	C77.1
Retroperitoneal	C77.2
Liver	C78.7
Bone	C79.51
Lung	C33
Brain	C71.9

Syndromes	Code
Malignant Neoplasm Pancreas, Produce Insulin, Somatostatin & Glucagon	C25.4
Islets of Langerhans	C25.4
Carcinoid Syndrome	E34.0
Zollinger-Ellison Syndrome	E16.4
Sweet's Syndrome	L98.2
MEN-1	E31.21

(See Pancreatic Polypeptide [PP] [Chapter 4] and Meal [Sham Feeding] Stimulation for Vagal Integrity [Chapter 6] for specific tests and CPT codes)

SOMATOSTATINOMA

Somatostatin (somatotropin release–inhibiting factor [SRIF]) is a tetradecapeptide that inhibits numerous endocrine and exocrine secretory functions. Almost all gut hormones that have been studied are inhibited by SRIF, including insulin, PP, glucagon, gastrin, secretin, gastric inhibitory polypeptide (GIP), and motilin. In addition to inhibition of the endocrine secretions, SRIF has direct effects on a number of target organs. For example, it is a potent inhibitor of basal and PG-stimulated gastric acid secretion. It also has marked effects on GI transit time, intestinal motility, and absorption of nutrients from the small intestine. The major effect in the small intestine appears to be a delay in the absorption of fat and reduced absorption of calcium.

WHAT TO LOOK FOR

Distinguishing Signs and Symptoms

The salient features of the somatostatinoma syndrome are as follows:
- Diabetes
- Diarrhea/steatorrhea
- Gallbladder disease (cholelithiasis and dysmotility)
- Hypochlorhydria
- Weight loss

Diagnostic Markers

Plasma Somatostatin-Like Immunoreactivity
The mean somatostatin-like immunoreactivity (SLI) concentration in patients with pancreatic somatostatinoma was 50 times higher than normal (range, 1–250 times). Intestinal somatostatinomas, however, present differently and have only slightly elevated or normal SLI concentrations **(Table 1-10).**

Table 1-10. Comparison of Pancreatic and Intestinal Somatostatinoma

Pancreatic Somatostatinoma	Intestinal Somatostatinoma
SLI 50x higher than normal (range, 1–250 times)	SLI slightly elevated or normal
75% of patients have diabetes	11% of patients have diabetes
Tumors are large and destroy part of pancreas	Tumors are relatively small
59% of patients have gallbladder disease	27% of patients have gallbladder disease
Diarrhea and steatorrhea are common	Diarrhea and steatorrhea are rare
Weight loss in one third of patients	Weight loss in one fifth of patients
Acid secretion inhibited in 87% of patients	Acid secretion inhibited in 12% of patients
	Café-au-lait spots
	Neurofibromatosis
	Paroxysmal hypertension

THE NEXT STEP

Diabetes Mellitus

When pancreatic and intestinal tumors result in diabetes, the diabetes is relatively mild and can usually be controlled by diet with or without oral hypoglycemic agents or by small doses of insulin. It is not clear, however, whether the differential inhibition of insulin and diabetogenic hormones can explain the usually mild degree of diabetes and the rarity of ketoacidosis in patients with somatostatinoma. Replacement of functional islet cell tissue by pancreatic tumor may be another reason for the development of diabetes in most patients with pancreatic somatostatinoma, contrasting with the low incidence of diabetes in patients with intestinal tumors. Pancreatic tumors are usually large and therefore destroy substantial portions of the organ.

Gallbladder Disease

The high incidence of gallbladder disease in patients with somatostatinoma and the absence of such an association in any other islet cell tumor suggest a causal relation between gallbladder disease and somatostatinoma. Infusion of somatostatin into normal human subjects has been shown to inhibit gallbladder emptying, suggesting that somatostatin-mediated inhibition of gallbladder emptying (dysmotility) may cause the observed high rate of gallbladder disease in patients with somatostatinoma. This theory is supported by the observation of massively dilated gallbladders without stones or other pathology in patients with somatostatin-secreting tumors.

Diarrhea and Steatorrhea

Diarrhea consisting of 3 to 10 frequently foul-smelling stools per day and/or steatorrhea of 20 to 76 g of fat per 24 hours is common in patients with pancreatic somatostatinoma, even with a controlled amount of fat in the diet. This could result from the effects of high levels of somatostatin within the pancreas serving as a paracrine mediator to inhibit exocrine secretion or, alternatively, from duct obstruction caused by the somatostatinoma. In some cases, the severity of diarrhea and steatorrhea parallels the course of the disease, worsening as the tumor advances and metastatic disease spreads and improving after tumor resection. Somatostatin has been shown to inhibit the pancreatic secretion of proteolytic enzymes, water, bicarbonate, and gallbladder motility. In addition, it inhibits the absorption of lipids. All but 1 patient with diarrhea and steatorrhea have had high plasma somatostatin concentrations. The rarity of diarrhea and/or steatorrhea in patients with intestinal somatostatinomas may result from the lower SLI levels seen in patients with that condition.

Hypochlorhydria

Infusion of somatostatin has been shown to inhibit gastric acid secretion in human subjects. Thus, hypochlorhydria in patients with somatostatinoma, in the absence of gastric mucosal abnormalities, is likely to result from elevated somatostatin concentrations. Basal and stimulated acid secretion was inhibited in 87% of patients with pancreatic tumors tested but in only 12% of patients with intestinal tumors.

Weight Loss

Weight loss ranging from 9 to 21 kg over several months occurred in one third of patients with pancreatic tumors and one fifth of patients with intestinal tumors. The weight loss may relate to malabsorption and diarrhea, but in small intestinal tumors, anorexia, abdominal pain, and yet unexplained reasons may be relevant.

Associated Endocrine Disorders

Approximately 50% of all patients have other endocrinopathies in addition to their somatostatinoma. Occurrence of MEN-1 has been recognized in patients with islet cell tumors, and MEN-2 or MEN-3 syndromes are present in association with pheochromocytomas and neurofibromatosis, respectively. It seems that an additional dimension of the duct-associated tumors is MEN-2. Secretion of different hormones by the same islet cell tumor, sometimes resulting in two distinct clinical disorders, is now being recognized with increasing frequency. These possibilities should be considered during endocrine workups of patients with islet cell tumors and their relatives.

Tumor Location

Of the reported primary tumors, 60% were found in the pancreas and 40% in the duodenum or jejunum. Of the pancreatic tumors, 50% were located in the head, and 25% in the tail, and the remaining tumors either infiltrated the whole pancreas or were found in the body. Regarding extrapancreatic locations, approximately 50% originate in the duodenum, approximately 50% originate in the ampulla, and rarely one is found in the jejunum. Thus, approximately 60% of somatostatinomas originate in the upper intestinal tract, probably a consequence of the relatively large number of delta (somatostatin) cells in this region.

Tumor Size

Somatostatinomas tend to be large, similar to glucagonomas but unlike insulinomas and gastrinomas, which, as a rule, are small. Within the intestine, tumors tend to be smaller than somatostatinomas located elsewhere. Symptoms associated with somatostatinomas and glucagonomas are less pronounced and probably do not develop until very high blood levels of the respective hormones have been attained. As a result, somatostatinomas and glucagonomas are likely to be diagnosed late in the course of the disease.

Incidence of Malignancy

Eighty percent (80%) of patients with pancreatic somatostatinomas had metastases at diagnosis, and 50% with intestinal tumors had evidence of metastatic disease. Metastasis to the liver is most frequent, and regional lymph node involvement and metastases to bone are less so. Thus, in approximately 70% of cases, metastatic disease is present at diagnosis. This is similar to the high incidence of malignancy in glucagonoma and in gastrinoma, but it is distinctly different from the low incidence of malignant insulinoma. The high prevalence of metastatic disease in somatostatinoma also may be a consequence of late diagnosis but apparently is not dependent on the tissue of origin.

Somatostatin-Containing Tumors Outside the GI Tract

Somatostatin has been found in many tissues outside the GI tract. Prominent among those are the hypothalamic and extrahypothalamic regions of the brain, the peripheral nervous system (including the sympathetic adrenergic ganglia), and the C cells of the thyroid gland. Not surprisingly, therefore, high concentrations of somatostatin have been found in tumors originating from these tissues. Some patients exhibited the clinical somatostatinoma syndrome.

Elevated plasma SLI concentrations also have been reported in patients with small cell lung cancer. In one patient with metastatic bronchial oat cell carcinoma, the tumor caused Cushing's syndrome, diabetes, diarrhea, steatorrhea, anemia, and weight loss, and the patient had a plasma SLI concentration 20 times greater than normal. A patient with a bronchogenic carcinoma presenting with diabetic ketoacidosis and high levels of SLI (>5000 pg/mL) has been reported. Pheochromocytomas and catecholamine-producing extra-adrenal paragangliomas are other examples of endocrine tumors that produce and secrete somatostatin in addition to other hormonally active substances. One fourth of 37 patients with pheochromocytomas had elevated SLI levels.

Tumors are identified as somatostatinomas by the demonstration of elevated tissue concentrations of SLI and/or prevalence of D cells by immunocytochemistry or demonstration of elevated plasma SLI concentrations. Thus, events leading to the diagnosis of somatostatinoma usually occur in reverse order. In other islet cell tumors, the clinical symptoms and signs usually suggest the diagnosis, which then is established by demonstration of diagnostically elevated blood hormone levels, following which efforts are undertaken to localize the tumors.

The diagnosis of somatostatinoma at a time when blood SLI concentrations are normal or only marginally elevated, however, requires reliable provocative tests. Increased plasma SLI concentrations have been reported after intravenous infusion of tolbutamide and arginine, and decreased SLI concentrations have been observed after intravenous infusion of diazoxide. Arginine is a well-established stimulant for normal D cells and thus is unlikely to differentiate between normal and supranormal somatostatin secretion. The same may be true for diazoxide, which has been shown to decrease SLI secretion from normal dog pancreas as well as in patients with somatostatinoma. Tolbutamide stimulates SLI release from normal dog and rat pancreas, but no change was found in circulating SLI concentrations of three healthy human subjects after intravenous injection of 1 g of tolbutamide. Therefore, at present, tolbutamide appears to be a candidate for a provocative agent in the diagnosis of somatostatinoma, but its reliability must be established in a greater number of patients and controls. Until then, it may be necessary to measure plasma SLI concentrations during routine workups for postprandial dyspepsia and gallbladder disorders, for diabetes in patients without a family history, and for unexplained steatorrhea, because these findings can be early signs of somatostatinoma. Tolbutamide infusions are considered to have significant risks and should only be administered under strict medical observation.

ICD-10 CODE: Achlorhydria K31.83

ICD-10 CODE: Diabetes
    Type 1 (not specified as uncontrolled) E10.9
    Type 1 (uncontrolled) E10.65
    Type 2 (or unspecified) E11.9
    Type 2 (uncontrolled) E11.65

ICD-10 CODE: Diarrhea R19.7

ICD-10 CODE: Functional Diarrhea K59.1

ICD-10 CODE: Gallbladder Disease K82.9
    Congenital Q44.1

ICD-10 CODE: Hypochlorhydria K30
    Neurotic F45.8
    Psychogenic F45.8

ICD-10: CODE: Hypoglycemia E16.1

ICD-10 CODE: Malignant Neoplasm of the Pancreas, Producing Insulin, Somatostatin, and Glucagon
Islets of Langerhans C25.4

ICD-10 CODE: Malignant Neoplasm of the Intestine
Intestinal tract, part unspecified C26.0
Uncertain behavior, neoplasm of the intestine D37.2

ICD-10 CODE: Reactive Hypoglycemia NOS E16.2

ICD-10 CODE: Somatostatinoma C25.4

ICD-10 CODES for Primary pNETS Tumor Sites

Sites	Malignant	Benign	Uncertain Behavior	Unspecified
Ampulla	C24.1	D13.4/D13.5	D37.6	D40.0
Duodenum	C17.0	D13.2	D37.2	D49.0
Jejunum	C17.1	D13.2	D37.2	D49.0
Pancreas	C25.9	D13.6	D37.8	D49.0
Body	C25.1	D13.6	D37.8	D49.0
Head	C25.0	D13.6	D37.8	D49.0
Islet cell	C25.4	D13.7	D37.8	D49.0
Neck	C25.7	D13.6	D37.8	D49.0
Tail	C25.2	D13.6	D37.8	D49.0

ICD-10 CODES for pNETs Metastatic Sites and Syndromes

Sites	Malignant
Supraclavicular	C77.0
Abdominal	C77.2
Mediastinal	C77.1
Retroperitoneal	C77.2
Liver	C78.7
Bone	C79.51
Lung	C33
Brain	C71.9

Syndromes	Code
Malignant Neoplasm Pancreas, Produce Insulin, Somatostatin & Glucagon	C25.4
Islets of Langerhans	C25.4
Carcinoid Syndrome	E34.0
Zollinger-Ellison Syndrome	E16.4
Sweet's Syndrome	L98.2
MEN-1	E31.21

(See Somatostatin [Somatotropin Release–Inhibiting Factor (SRIF)] [Chapter 4] for specific tests and CPT codes)

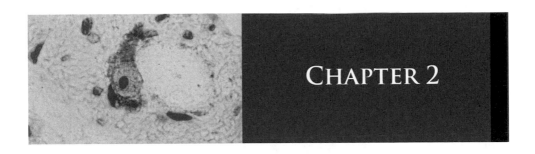

CHAPTER 2

NEUROENDOCRINE TUMORS IN CHILDREN AND YOUNG ADULTS BY M. SUE O'DORISIO, MD, PHD

NEUROENDOCRINE TUMORS
A COMPREHENSIVE GUIDE TO DIAGNOSIS AND MANAGEMENT

NEUROENDOCRINE TUMORS (NETS) IN KIDS

The rationale for separate discussion of non-familial neuroendocrine tumors in children and in young adults under the age of 30 is based on the following observations:

1) neuroendocrine tumors are as common as neuroblastoma in the birth-29 year age group[1]
2) neuroendocrine tumors, especially those tumors previously classified as carcinoid, are diagnosed four to nine years after the first symptoms[2];
3) with the exception of appendiceal tumors, nearly 40% of neuroendocrine tumors in children and young adults are metastatic at diagnosis[1];
4) adolescents and young adults with cancer have poorer overall survival than any other age group in the United States[3].

Neuroendocrine tumors arise from either the diffuse neuroendocrine system or the neural crest as outlined in the table below.

Diffuse Neuroendocrine System	Neural crest
Multiple endocrine neoplasia 1 & 2	Neuroblastoma
Neuroendocrine tumors of breast, lung, intestine, pancreas	Pheochromocytoma
Small cell carcinoma of cervix, ovary	Paraganglioma
Unknown primary NET	Peripheral primitive neuroectodermal tumor

According to the SEER database, every neuroendocrine tumor observed in adults also occurs in children. The incidence increases with age and nearly 90% of NETs in the 0-29 year age group are diagnosed over the age of 21. However, the tendency to late diagnosis, after metastases to the liver or bones, suggests that more than half of NETs diagnosed in this age group actually occur prior to age 21. The adrenal is the most common site for neural crest tumors; 65% of neuroblastomas and >85% of pheochromocytomas arise from the adrenal.

NEUROENDOCRINE TUMORS

Because neuroendocrine tumors are both rare and slow growing, the diagnosis of a NET is highly dependent upon recognition of signs and symptoms. While "non-functioning" pancreatic tumors may be asymptomatic, all other neuroendocrine tumors will have both symptoms and abnormal biomarkers. As described in Chapter 1, the symptoms are often non-specific, including weight loss, fatigue, intermittent flushing, cough, wheezing, vague abdominal pain, and diarrhea. The specific biomarkers used to screen for NETs in children are the same as in adults; however, caution should be taken when interpreting the levels as age specific normal values have not been determined for all NET biomarkers. Age-specific peptide levels are shown in Table 1 for a few key biomarkers[4].

Table 2-1. Plasma neuropeptide levels in normal children.

Age (n)	IGF-1, ND = < 150 pg/mL	VIP, ND = < 30 pg/mL	Somatosta-tin, ND = < 20 pg/mL	GRP, ND = < 100 pg/mL	Sub P, ND = < 20 pg/mL	Pancreast-atin** ND = < 20 pg/mL	NPY, ND = < 50 pg/mL
Cord blood (6)*	90 ± 44	ND	ND	124.5 ± 40, 4 ND	45 ± 35, 1 ND	109 ± 68, 1 ND	70 ± 32, 4 ND
0 - 11 months (2)†	43.5 ± 29	52 ± 16	41 ± 30, 1 ND	ND	81 ± 7	77 ± 42	ND
12 - 35 months (3)*	53 ± 14.5	58 ± 14	25 ± 9, 2 ND	ND	94 ± 49	77 ± 55, 1 ND	ND
3 - 5 years (10)*	120 ± 45	59 ± 15	28.8 ± 15	109 ± 21.5, 7 ND	108 ± 50	50 ± 23, 2 ND	51 ± 2.5, 9 ND
6 - 11 years (15)*	340 ± 166	54 ± 22, 2 ND	30 ± 14, 8 ND	234 ± 415, 12 ND	110 ± 65, 2 ND	47 ± 27, 3 ND	51 ± 3.4, 13 ND
12 - 21 years (11)*	401 ± 179	56 ± 12, 1 ND	29 ± 17, 8 ND	111 ± 27.5, 8 ND	55 ± 38, 4 ND	47 ± 24.5, 2 ND	ND

ND = non-detectable
* = Mean ± S.D.
† = Mean ± range.
IGF-1 = Insulin-Like Growth Factor 1; VIP = Vasoactive Intestinal Polypeptide; GRP = Gastrin Releasing Peptide (Bombesin);
Sub P = Substance P; NPY = Neuropeptide Y. Neuropeptide data from the Ohio State University Reference Lab.
**Pancreastatin levels differ from ISI's values by a factor of five.

The distribution of primary neuroendocrine tumors varies from those in adults[1]. The three most common locations for diffuse neuroendocrine system tumors in the 0-29 year age group are lung, appendix and breast with midgut, ovary, and unknown primary NETs close behind as shown in Figure 1.

Table 2-2. The distribution of 1,073 malignant tumors by common primary sites for 0-29 year olds, nine standard SEER registries 1975 - 2006.

Location of Primary	% Distribution
Lung	28%
Breast	18%
Appendix	18%
Hindgut	9%
Unknown primary site	5%
Midgut	5%
Gonads	5%
Foregut	4%
Thyroid gland	4%
Cervix	4%

Neuroendocrine tumor is the most common childhood malignancy arising in the lung[5]. NETs should be considered in any young person who has a culture negative pneumonia and especially in the case of recurrent, culture negative pneumonia. NET biomarker levels should be measured and a biopsy obtained as outlined in the following diagnostic algorithm.

NET biomarker levels should be obtained at the time of a lung biopsy and can be used to follow the course of disease if the biopsy demonstrates neuroendocrine tumor.

The appendix is the second most common site for a neuroendocrine tumor in a child or young adult and it is most often an incidental finding; however, as noted in Table 1-2 of Chapter 1, 35% of appendiceal NETs metastasize. Therefore, the major question in a child or young adult is whether or not to perform a right hemicolectomy and at the present time, the recommendation is the same as for adults, namely, a tumor >2 cm diameter or invasion of peri-appendiceal fat warrants hemicolectomy. A surgical consult should be obtained for any child whose tumor is >1.5 cm in greatest diameter or the pathology report suggests any invasion. Recommended follow-up for appendiceal NET in a child is measurement of plasma pancreastatin, chromogranin A, and serotonin every three months for 1 year, every 6 months for 2 additional years and yearly thereafter until symptom free with a normal peptide profile for 10 years post appendectomy. The role of serial plasma NKA determination has not yet been evaluated in children.

Neuroendocrine tumor is most often an unexpected finding in a breast biopsy. In this case a full metastatic workup, including full screening for peptide or other biomarkers should be undertaken prior to removal of the primary lesion. Additionally, the tumor should be stained for biomarkers to determine the best biomarkers to utilize in follow-up which will be as outlined above for appendiceal tumors.

Workup of midgut and other gastroenteropancreatic tumors in children is slightly different from that of adults, mostly due to the frequency of constipation and virally induced diarrhea in the younger age group. Furthermore, flushing is very common in children and young adults, making the differential diagnosis more difficult in this age group and emphasizing the need for recognition of the incidence of NETs in this age group.

NEUROBLASTOMA

Neuroblastoma has a higher incidence than other neuroendocrine tumors in the 0-10 year age group; it usually presents as a mass. Peptide and catecholamine levels can aid in diagnosis, can provide prognostic information, and when positive, can serve as a sensitive and specific disease monitor. High VMA/HVA in a 24 hr urine is a diagnostic criteria; catecholamines are high in patients with hypertension. VIP is high in patients with diarrhea and this is a good prognostic indicator while NPY is a sensitive marker of disease recurrence in children with minimal residual disease. Biopsy of lymph node, primary tumor and a bone marrow are necessary for diagnosis. PET/CT using ^{68}Ga-PET/CT and/or SPECT/CT employing ^{123}I-MIBG both provide comprehensive imaging technique for staging. Of note, the radiation dose produced by a ^{68}Ga is one half the dose of an OctreoScan® in children.

GASTRINOMA

Diarrhea is extremely common and peptic ulcer disease is also common in children. Gastrinoma is extremely rare in children, but has reported as early as 7 years of age. Normal fasting gastrin levels are similar in children and adults, making this an easy and extremely useful test. However, chronic use of proton pump inhibitors (PPI) can significantly raise gastrin levels and thus should be discontinued for at least 72 hours prior to obtaining a gastrin level, and may require up to 4 weeks, depending on the duration of PPI use. **(See Table 1-4)**

INSULINOMA/NESIDIOBLASTOSIS

Nesidioblastosis is the result of an overactive pancreas (hypertrophy and hyperplasia of the islet cells) and most often presents at birth as hypoglycemia unresponsive to feeding or IV glucose. This most often resolves with close follow-up and octreotide therapy, but may resurface when these children reach puberty. Insulin and C-peptide levels are measured in blood and normal levels are similar to adults.

MULTIPLE ENDOCRINE NEOPLASIA

MEN 1 occurs in parathyroid, pancreas and pituitary. MEN 2a occurs in parathyroid, thyroid (medullary thyroid carcinoid MCT) and adrenal (pheochromocytoma), while MEN 2b includes MCT, pheochromocytoma and neural crest tumors. Family history and blood pressure measurements are the most important screening tools. Children can be tested and diagnosis made as early as 4 years of age with blood calcitonin levels; the pentagastrin stimulation test is available, but rarely performed. Urine catecholamines are also important and require a 24 hour urine test. Age at which thyroidectomy is recommended for children with MEN 2a or MEN 2b is controversial[6].

PHEOCHROMOCYTOMA

Pheochromocytoma is associated with MEN 2a and 2b, von Hippel-Landau, and neuro-fibromatosis. With the peak incidence between 9 and 12 years of age (VHL), nearly 10% of all pheochromocytomas occur in children and 10% of these are malignant. Headaches, palpitations, diaphoresis, and hypertension are the most common symptoms. Diagnostic testing should include twenty four hour urine for creatinine, VMA, catecholamines and metanephrines plus plasma free metanephrine and normeta-nephrines and chromogranin A. Since pheochromocytoma can be seen in adolescents and young adults, drug interference with metanephrine testing should be ruled out with a careful medication and illicit drug history. False positive metanephrines can be caused by: buspirone, benzodiazepines, methyldopa, labetalol, tricyclic antidepressants; levodopa, ethanol, amphetamines, sotalol, and chlorpromazine.

PARAGANGLIOMA

Extra-adrenal phenochromocytomas comprise nearly 15 – 25% of pheochromocytomas in children and are characteristic of VHL syndrome. Symptoms are the same as for pheochromocytoma.

MUNCHAUSEN'S SYNDROME BY PROXY

Diarrhea, flushing, sweating, fatigue are hallmark symptoms of neuroendocrine tumors; however, each of these symptoms is common in normal, healthy children associated with viral infections, topical exposures, and allergies. These symptoms can be induced quite easily by a parent, relative, or guardian. Fictitious diarrhea can be induced with laxatives and should be included in the screening process. Ricins cause overall irritation of the GI tract, whereas, castor oil will induce vomiting as well as some GI upset. These can be measured in the stool along with pH and stool electrolyte.

Flushing is seldom witnessed by medical personnel. It can be caused by allergic reactions, serotonin uptake inhibitors such as Zoloft or Prozac, and even by overuse of niacin (vitamin B3).

Sweating is likewise difficult to provoke in an office setting and thus is seldom witnessed by medical personnel. The sweating of Hodgkin's Disease is easily distinguished and most often occurs at night and is described as drenching.

Fatigue is a soft symptom that is very difficult to evaluate, but is most often the result of too little sleep. Children and adolescents should receive 8-10 hours each night, significantly more than most adults require.

An overly solicitous parent who is extremely knowledgeable about medical terminology and procedures along with a history of multiple professional caregivers for the child should raise the possibility of Munchausen's by proxy in the differential diagnosis. The availability of medical information on the internet has contributed to this explosion of medical knowledge, but in the case of Munchausen's, important details may be missing from the child's history that rule against a neuroendocrine tumors as the true cause of the symptoms.

References

1. Navalkele, P., et al., *Incidence, survival, and prevalence of neuroendocrine tumors versus neuroblastoma in children and young adults: nine standard SEER registries, 1975-2006.* Pediatr Blood Cancer, 2011. 56(1): p. 50-7.

2. Vinik, A.I. and A.R. Moattari, *Treatment of endocrine tumors of the pancreas.* Endocrinol Metab Clin North Am, 1989. 18(2): p. 483-518.

3. Bleyer, A., et al., *Relative lack of conditional survival improvement in young adults with cancer.* Semin Oncol, 2009. 36(5): p. 460-7.

4. O'Dorisio, M.S., M. Hauger, and T.M. O'Dorisio, *Age-dependent levels of plasma neuropeptides in normal children.* Regul.Pept., 2002. 109(1-3): p. 189-192.

5. Gustafsson, B.I., et al., *Bronchopulmonary neuroendocrine tumors.* Cancer, 2008. 113(1): p. 5-21.

6. Calva, D., et al., *When is prophylactic thyroidectomy indicated for patients with the RET codon 609 mutation?* Ann Surg Oncol, 2009. 16(8): p. 2237-44.

7. Howlader N, Noone AM, Krapcho M, Neyman N, Aminou R, Altekruse SF, Kosary CL, Ruhl J, Tatalovich Z, Cho H, Mariotto A, Eisner MP, Lewis DR, Chen HS, Feuer EJ, Cronin KA (eds). SEER Cancer Statistics Review, 1975-2009 (Vintage 2009 Populations), National Cancer Institute. Bethesda, MD, http://seer.cancer.gov/csr/1975_2009_pops09/, based on November 2011 SEER data submission.

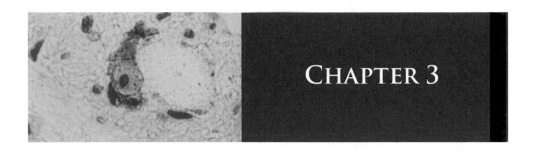

CHAPTER 3

CLINICAL PRESENTATIONS AND THEIR SYNDROMES, INCLUDING ICD-10 CODES

NEUROENDOCRINE TUMORS
A COMPREHENSIVE GUIDE TO DIAGNOSIS AND MANAGEMENT

CLINICAL PRESENTATIONS AND THEIR SYNDROMES, INCLUDING ICD-10 CODES

This chapter highlights the clinical manifestations related to the GEP neuroendocrine system for the symptoms and syndromes shown below. Guidance is provided for each syndrome, including possible causes, distinguishing signs and symptoms to look for and, finally, recommended hormone/peptide testing and dynamic testing protocols, with imaging where applicable, as the next step of treatment for each.

The frequency of clinical manifestations presents as follows:

Flushing	84%
Diarrhea	79%
Hypertension*	50%
Bronchoconstriction	17%
Heart disease*	<10%
Myopathy	7%
Pigmentation	5%
Arthropathy	5%
Hyper-hypoglycemia	<1%
Ulcer disease	<1%
Dermopathy	<1%

*Note that the incidence of right-sided valvular heart disease has markedly decreased in the last two decades since the widespread use of somatostatin analogs. However, the incidence of hypertension has increased over this same time period.

FLUSHING

Flushing, a cardinal symptom of carcinoid tumors, occurs in a variety of other conditions. A good rule of thumb is if the flushing is "wet" (accompanied by sweating), it is due to a cause other than carcinoid. **Table 3-1** lists the differential diagnosis and the features that help distinguish flushing caused by carcinoid from flushing associated with other conditions.

Table 3-1. Features Associated With Various Flushing Syndromes

Flushing Syndrome	Associated Features
Carcinoid	Diarrhea, wheezing
MCT	Mass in neck, family history
Pheochromocytoma	Paroxysmal hypertension, tachycardia
Diabetes	Autonomic neuropathy/chlorpropamide
Menopause	Cessation of menses
Autonomic epilepsy	Diencephalic seizures
Panic syndrome	Phobias, anxiety
Mastocytosis	Dyspepsia, peptic ulcer, dermatographia
Drugs	Niacin, alcohol, calcium channel blockers
Idiopathic	Diagnosis by exclusion
Cardiac	Angina in women, mitral valve prolapse

WHAT TO LOOK FOR

Distinguishing Signs and Symptoms

There are two varieties of flushing in carcinoid syndrome:
1. Midgut carcinoid: The flush usually is faint pink to red in color and involves the face and upper trunk as far as the nipple line. The flush is initially provoked by alcohol and food containing tyramine (e.g., blue cheese, chocolate, aged or cured sausage, red wine). With time, the flush may occur spontaneously and without provocation. It usually lasts only a few minutes and may occur many times per day. It generally does not leave permanent discoloration.
2. Foregut tumors: The flush often is more intense, of longer duration, and purplish in hue. It is frequently followed by telangiectasia and involves not only the upper trunk but may also affect the limbs. The limbs may become acrocyanotic, and the appearance of the nose resembles that of rhinophyma. The skin of the face often thickens, and assumes leonine facies resembling that seen in leprosy and acromegaly.

THE NEXT STEP

Other Clinical Conditions

Because flushing cannot always be attributed to carcinoid syndrome, as mentioned previously, the differential diagnosis of flushing is extremely important and includes the following:
- Postmenopausal state
- Simultaneous ingestion of chlorpropamide and alcohol
- Panic attacks
- MCT
- Autonomic epilepsy
- Autonomic neuropathy
- Mastocytosis

- Ganglioneuromas
- Carotid body tumors
- Pheochromocytomas

Hormones and Peptides

Measure the levels of the following hormones and peptides ascribed to flushing in carcinoid syndrome:
- 5-HIAA (Plasma or urine)
- Calcitonin
- Gastrin
- Gastrin-releasing peptide (GRP)
- Kinins
- Motilin
- Neurokinin A (NKA)
- Neurotensin
- Prostaglandins
- Serotonin (5-HT)
- Somatostatin
- Substance P
- Vasoactive neuropeptides (serotonin, dopamine, histamine)
- Vasoactive Intestinal Polypeptide (VIP)

Several tests are used to identify the cause of flushing in carcinoid syndrome **(Table 3-2)**.

Table 3-2. Tests to Identify Cause of Flushing

Clinical Condition	Tests
Carcinoid	Plasma or Urine 5-HIAA, 5-HTP, substance P, CGRP, CgA
MCT	Calcitonin, calcium infusion, RET protooncogene
Pheochromocytoma	VMA, epinephrine, norepinephrine, glucagon stimulation,[131]I-MIBG
Diabetic autonomic neuropathy	Heart rate variability, 2-hour PP, glucose
Menopause	FSH
Epilepsy	Electroencephalogram
Panic syndrome	Pentagastrin/ACTH
Mastocytosis	Plasma histamine, plasma or urine tryptase
Hypomastia, mitral prolapse	Cardiac echogram

ICD-10 CODE: Autonomic Epilepsy
Without mention of intractable epilepsy G40.101 or G40.109
With intractable epilepsy G40.111 or G40.119

ICD-10 CODE: Carcinoid Syndrome E34.0

ICD-10 CODE: Diabetes, Autonomic Neuropathy
Diabetes with neurological manifestations,
  Type I (juvenile type), not stated as uncontrolled E10.44
Diabetes with neurological manifestations,
  Type II or unspecified type, not stated as uncontrolled E11.40
  Amyotrophy E10.44 or E11.44
  Gastroparalysis K31.84
  Use additional code to identify manifestations, as Gastroparesis K31.84
Diabetic
  Mononeuropathy E10.41 or E11.41
  Neurogenic arthropathy E10.618 or E11.618
  Peripheral Autonomic Neuropathy E10.43 or E11.43
  Polyneuropathy E10.42 or E11.42
Diabetes with neurological manifestations,
  Type II or unspecified type, uncontrolled E11.65
Diabetes with neurological manifestations,
  Type I (juvenile type), uncontrolled E10.65

ICD-10 CODE: Flushing R23.2

ICD-10 CODE: Hypomastia (Congenital) Q38.8

ICD-10 CODE: Mastocytosis Q82.2
Malignant mast cell tumors C96.2
Systemic D47.0

ICD-10 CODE: Medullary Carcinoma Thyroid
With amyloid stroma
  Specified site, thyroid C73
  Unspecified site C73
With lymphoid stroma
Malignant thyroid C73
  Uncertain behavior, neoplasm of thyroid D44.0
  Disorders of thryocalcitonin secretion E07.0

ICD-10 CODE: Mitral Prolapse I34.0

ICD-10 CODE: Panic Attack F41.0

ICD-10 CODE: Pheochromocytoma
Malignant
  Specified site–see Neoplasm by site, malignant
  Unspecified site C74.10
Benign
  Specified site–see Neoplasm by site, benign
  Unspecified site D35.00

(See Flushing Syndrome Tests [Chapter 5] for specific tests and individual CPT codes)

DIARRHEA

Watery diarrhea syndrome (WDHHA), which is caused by a pancreatic islet cell tumor, was first identified by Verner and Morrison in 1958. As implied by its name, the primary characteristic is watery diarrhea. A critical distinguishing difference from ZE is the absence of hyperacidity and the marked presence of hypokalemia. Diarrhea in ZE improves with inhibition of acid secretion, whereas in WDHHA it does not. The WDHHA usually begins with intermittent diarrhea, but as the tumor grows, the episodic diarrhea becomes continuous and persists despite fasting (i.e., it is secretory, not malabsorptive). Hypercalcemia occurs in WDHHA because of direct effects of VIP on bone. It is important to differentiate this cause of hypercalcemia from the hypercalcemia caused by excess PTH release from parathyroid glands seen in the sporadic (usually caused by adenomas) or familial (usually the result of hyperplastic glands) forms of hyperthyroidism. Factitious diarrhea can be difficult to distinguish and requires the demonstration of an osmolar gap. If 2x [Na+ +K+] is less than stool osmolality (i.e., osmotic gap), search for idiogenic osmoles.

The following are characteristics of secretory diarrhea:
- Large-volume stools
- Persists during fasting
- 2 x [Na+ +K+] = stool osmolality

The following are characteristics of osmotic diarrhea:
- Small volume (<1 L/d)
- Disappears with fasting

WHAT TO LOOK FOR

Distinguishing Signs and Symptoms

- Profuse diarrhea with the appearance of weak tea
- Presence of marked hypokalemia and hyperchloremic acidosis
- Initial intermittent diarrhea, becoming continuous as tumor grows
- Secretory nature of diarrhea (i.e., does not disappear even after fasting for 48 hours)
- Absence of gastric hyperacidity (a major feature distinguishing WDHHA from ZE)
- Atrophic gastritis or pernicious anemia or gastric carcinoid type 1
- Hypochlorhydria resulting from the gastric inhibitory effect of VIP
- Secretion of HCO3 and causes life-threatening loss of electrolytes into the stool
- Increased intestinal motility as well as secretion adding to the diarrhea
- Hypercalcemia not due to PTH or PTHrp
- Hyperglycemia or abnormal glucose tolerance
- Dilation of the gallbladder
- Flushing
- Weight loss
- Colic

THE NEXT STEP

Patients with watery diarrhea are often severely dehydrated, and their fluid balance and electrolytes should be corrected before specific diagnostic tests are initiated, except for evaluation of stool electrolytes and osmolarity.

Diagnostic tests should be selected to:
- Exclude atrophic gastritis, pernicious anemia, and gastric carcinoid
- Exclude use of proton pump inhibitors
- Exclude ZE
- Determine the probability of a pancreatic-based source of watery diarrhea (VIP, Pancreatic Polypeptide(PP), MCT, CT, and OctreoScan®)
- Eliminate other syndromes masquerading as WDHHA and producing similar symptoms

Hormones and Peptides

Vasoactive intestinal polypeptide is the primary peptide produced by the majority of pancreatic tumors (VIPomas) causing WDHHA, but substance P, PP, calcitonin gene–related peptide (CGRP) and thyrocalcitonin (TCT) have also been implicated in NET-related diarrhea. Because VIP is also produced by neural cells, elevated levels of other GI and pancreatic hormones and peptides may be markers for establishing the presence of a pancreatic tumor associated with diarrhea. WDHHA in children is most commonly due to a nonpancreatic NET such as neuroblastoma. Occasionally, adults with pheochromocytomas may secrete VIP, which releases prolactin and is a vasodilator in the corpora cavernosa. However, this does not appear to be part of the clinical syndrome **(Fig. 3-1)**.

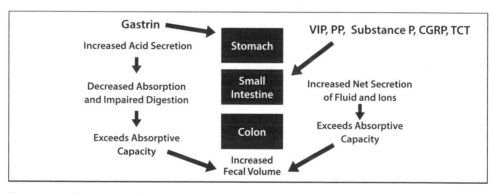

Figure 3-1. Pathogenesis of Endocrine Diarrhea

After mechanical causes have been ruled out, use the following ICD-10 codes:
ICD-10 CODE: Achlorhydria K31.83

ICD-10 CODE: Diarrhea R19.7

ICD-10 CODE: Functional K59.1

(See Table 1-1 for primary tumor sites and common metastatic tumor sites)
(See Diarrhea Syndrome Tests [Chapter 5] for specific tests and individual CPT codes)

Reference
1. Verner JV, Morrison AB. Islet cell tumor and a syndrome of refractory watery diarrhea and hypokalemia. *Am J Med.*1958; Sept;25(3):374-80.

Endocrine Hypertension

Up to 50% of individuals with hypertension are not controlled on their anti-hypertensive medications. While medication non-compliance is a common cause for poor control, many individuals will have a secondary cause for their elevated blood pressure, and many of these conditions are related to endocrine gland hyper- or hypofunction. A number of these conditions are described in further detail in this text.

Specific conditions to consider include:
- Hypo- and Hyperthyroidism
- Hyperparathyroidism
- Pheochromocytoma/Paraganglioma
- Carcinoid Syndrome
- Hyperaldosteronism
- Cushing's syndrome/Hypercortisolism
- Acromegaly
- Congenital adrenal hyperplasia

What to Look For

Distinguishing Signs and Symptoms
- Hypothyroidism: cold intolerance, fatigue, dry skin, brittle nails, constipation, depression, abnormal menses
- Hyperparathyroidism: hypercalcemia, kidney stones, abdominal pain, constipation, depression, polydipsia and polyuria, confusion
- Hyperthyroidism: heat intolerance, fatigue, oily skin and hair, frequent stooling, anxiety, palpitations, tremor. abnormal menses, eye discomfort and bulging eyes.
- Pheochromocytoma/Paraganglioma: palpitations, sweating, headaches, spells, orthostatic hypotension (see section on pheochromocytoma)
- Carcinoid syndrome, Flushing which is dry, diarrhea which persisits with fasting, pellagra like skin eruption, proximal muscle weakness and cardiopathy with dyspnea, edema and exercise intolerance
- Hyperaldosteronism: hypertension, hypokalemia, weakness, polydipsia and polyuria, tingling and tetany
- Cushing's syndrome/Hypercortisolism: obesity, facial flushing, moon facies, skin thinning, easy skin bruising, easy bleeding, proximal muscle weakness, wide/purple plapable striae, irritability, abnormal menses, supraclavicular and dorsocervical fat pad thickening
- Acromegaly: frontal bossing, carpal tunnel syndrome, palmar sweating, large hands and feet, changes in shoe, ring and/or hat size, prognathism
- Congenital adrenal hyperplasia: hirsutism, acne; Hispanic/Ashkenazi Jewish/Slavic background, abnormal menses

THE NEXT STEP

Hormones and Peptides

- Pancreastatin, Neurokinin A, Serotonin, CgA, Plasma 5HIAA
- Vasostatin 1 and 2
- TSH
- Free T4 and free T3
- PTH and PTH rp
- 24 hour urinary calcium and creatinine
- 25-hydroxy and 1:25 hydroxy vitamin D
- Plasma free fractionated metanephrines
- Urine fractionated metanephrines and catecholamines
- Basic metabolic panel with potassium
- Plasma aldosterone concentration
- Plasma renin activity or direct renin concentration
- 24 hour urine free cortisol and creatinine
- Late-night salivary cortisol
- ACTH
- Cortisol the morning after 1-mg of dexamethasone
- Growth hormone
- Insulin-like growth factor-1
- 17-hydroxy progesterone and progesterone

CONFIRMATORY/LOCALIZING TESTS

Hyperaldosteronism: 24 hour urine aldosterone after salt-loading or saline-suppression test, adrenal vein sampling

Cushing's syndrome/Hypercortisolism: Dexamethasone suppression testing, inferior petrosal sinus sampling

Acromegaly: oral glucose tolerance test

Congenital adrenal hyperplasia: ACTH stimulation testing

References
1. Calhoun DA, Jones D et al. Resistant Hypertension: Diagnosis, Evaluation and Treatment: A Scientific Statement from the American Heart Association Professional Education Committee of the Council for High Blood Pressure Research. *Circulation.* 2008; 117:e510-e526.
2. Young WF. Endocrine Hypertension. In: Melmed S, Polonsky KS, Larsen PR, Kronenberg HM, eds. Williams Textbook of Endocrinology, 12th ed. Philadelphia, PA: Elsevier Saunders; 2011: 545-577.
3. Vinik AI and Gonzales MR. New and emerging syndromes due to neuroendocrine tumors. Endocrinol Metab Clin North Am. 2011;40.1:19-63, vii.

(See for individual tests and CPT codes [Chapter 4] for specific tests and CPT codes and Syndromes [Chapter 5])

BRONCHOCONSTRICTION (WHEEZING)

Wheezing due to bronchospasm occurs in about one third of patients with carcinoid syndrome and in patients with mastocytosis.

WHAT TO LOOK FOR

Distinguishing Signs and Symptoms

Wheezing can be readily assessed at the bedside by asking the patient to breathe out as quickly as possible and listening to the trachea. Normally the wheezing is almost instantaneous, but with the expiratory bronchospasm in carcinoid and mastocytosis it is often prolonged. A test dose of octreotide acetate (100 µg) administered intravenously will relieve carcinoid bronchospasm. It is not known what effects octreotide has on asthma.

THE NEXT STEP

Lung function tests reveal a prolongation of forced expiratory volume in 1 second (FEV1), which needs to be distinguished from asthma and chronic airways obstructive disease. Refer the patient to a pulmonologist.

Hormones and Peptides

Wheezing is predominantly the result of the bronchoconstrictive effects of substance P, histamine, and possibly 5-HT.

ICD-10 CODE: Asthma
Unspecified J45.909
With status asthmaticus J45.902
With (acute) exacerbation J45.901

ICD-10 CODE: Bronchospasm J98.01

ICD-10 CODE: Carcinoid Syndrome E34.01

ICD-10 CODE: Wheezing R06.2

(See for individual tests and CPT codes [Chapter 4] for specific tests and CPT codes Carcinoid Follow-Up Profile & Bronchospasm Profile [Chapter 5])

CARCINOID HEART DISEASE

The prevalence and incidence of carcinoid heart disease has changed dramatically over the years particularly with the introduction of management of the comorbidities such as hypertension and the use of Somatostatin analogs. Earlier estimates of the prevalence of carcinoid heart disease were around 37% of patients(Vinik and Gonzales 19-63, vii). In a retrospective assessment of data collected from the medical charts of patients diagnosed with NETs who were treated with octreotide LAR at 36 sites in the United States during the period between October 31, 2000, and September 30, 2006 the prevalence of carcinoid heart disease and the impact of treatment was re-examined.

Medical records of 392 patients (186 women and 206 men) were reviewed for this study. Patients were stratified according to disease status: 106 patients (27%) did not exhibit CS, 260 patients (66%) exhibited CS at initial diagnosis, and 24 patients developed CS after the diagnosis of NET was established. Only 20 patients (5% of the total population) had evidence of carcinoid heart disease, all of whom had carcinoid syndrome. The presence of carcinoid heart disease was determined by echocardiogram or physical examination. The patients' charts demonstrated that 3 months after treatment with Octreotide began, 4 of the 20 patients no longer showed evidence of the condition and 4 patients showed improvement(Anthony and Vinik 987-94). Thus it appears that carcinoid heart disease may well be disappearing with the advent of treatment with Sandostatin and control of hypertension. Nonetheless, in patients who have dyspnea, exercise intolerance, fatigue and pedal edema and the presence of cardiac findings suggesting tricuspid or mitral valve disease and pulmonary hypertension with a serotonin level > 1000 ng/mL an echocardiogram should be done and if there is significant valvular disease consideration for valvular surgery should be considered.

References
1. Anthony L and Vinik AI. Evaluating the characteristics and the management of patients with neuroendocrine tumors receiving octreotide LAR during a 6-year period.Pancreas, 2011;40.7:987-94.
2. Vinik AI and Gonzales MR. New and emerging syndromes due to neuroendocrine tumors. Endocrinol Metab Clin North Am. 2011;40.1:19-63, vii.

DYSPEPSIA, PEPTIC ULCER

GASTRINOMA (ZOLLINGER-ELLISON SYNDROME)

Zollinger-Ellison syndrome is characterized by hyperacidity and gastric hypersecretion from an islet cell tumor (gastrinoma) of the pancreas or duodenum. Approximately 90% of gastrinomas are found in the "gastrinoma" triangle, an area bordered by the confluence of the cystic and common ducts superiorly, the mesenteric vessels medially, and the lateral sweep of the "C" loop of the duodenum laterally. A primary gastrinoma is rarely found in the liver or ovary, and even more rarely in a lymph node. These tumors may be associated with peptic perforation, obstruction, hemorrhage, and/or hyperacidity. Atrophic gastritis, pernicious anemia, gastric carcinoid, chronic proton pump inhibitor use, and diabetic gastropathy may produce spuriously high gastrin levels. A high gastrin level in the absence of diarrhea suggests atrophic gastritis. Secretory diarrhea in the presence of achlorhydria with normal gastrin levels suggests a VIPoma. Gastric pH measurement remains a valuable tool in distinguishing the causes of hypergastrinemia. Even though this measurement is easily performed, it is often overlooked. Gastric cell hyperplasia is another rare condition that can cause hypergastrinemia and hyperacidity. In all patients who have undergone peptic ulcer surgery with a Billroth II reconstruction, one must recognize the possibility of retained antrum syndrome.

WHAT TO LOOK FOR

Distinguishing Signs and Symptoms

- Highly elevated level of gastrin
- Diarrhea that responds to PPI

THE NEXT STEP

In conjunction with gastric acid measurement (gastric pH at the minimum), these syndromes may be distinguished, but provocative testing may be necessary.

Hormones and Peptides

Normal values of gastrin are less than 100 pg/mL. PPI will raise levels to 400 to 500 pg/mL. Fasting gastrin concentrations greater than 500 pg/mL in the presence of normal or excess gastric acid is suspicious of gastrinoma. Very high levels of greater than 1000 pg/mL may be pathognomonic of gastrinoma. Pernicious anemia and atrophic gastritis can produce gastrin levels greater than 1000 pg/mL, which should alert the clinician to the possibility of gastric carcinoid. Endoscopic pH measurements are essential to distinguish ZE from atrophic gastritis, type 1 gastric carcinoid, and pernicious anemia.

ICD-10 CODE: Dyspepsia and other specified disorders of function of stomach K30
  Peptic Ulcer, site unspecified K27.9

ICD-10 CODE: Peptic Ulcer
  Without obstruction K27.9
  With hemorrhage K27.4
    Without obstruction K27.2
    With obstruction K27.0
      And perforation K27.6
      Perforation (chronic) K27.5

ICD-10 CODE: Zollinger-Ellison/Gastrinoma E16.4
  Malignant
    Pancreas C25.4
    Specified site–see Neoplasm by site, malignant
    Unspecified site C25.9
  Benign
    Unspecified site D37.9
  Uncertain behavior, see Neoplasm

(See Table 1-1 for primary tumor sites and common metastatic tumor sites) (See Gastrin Test [Chapter 4] for specific tests and CPT codes)

Hypoglycemia

Hypoglycemia is a multifactorial disorder. Although the diagnosis of an insulin-secreting lesion of the pancreas is essential to successful management, it is critically important to rule out other causes of hypoglycemia.

What to Look For

Distinguishing Signs and Symptoms

- Organic hyperinsulinemia
    - Islet cell adenoma, carcinoma, hyperplasia, nesidioblastosis
- Fasting hypoglycemia
- Autoimmune with insulin antibodies
- Counter-regulatory hormone deficiency
    - Anterior pituitary insufficiency—GH, ACTH
    - Adrenocortical insufficiency
    - Severe hypothyroidism
    - Large non-islet tumor
    - Impaired hepatic function
    - Hepatocellular insufficiency
    - Ethanol/malnutrition
    - Sepsis
    - Specific enzymatic defects (childhood)
    - Impaired renal function
    - Substrate deficiency
    - Fanconi syndrome (renal loss)
    - Nursing
    - Severe inanition
    - Severe exercise
- Drug induced
    - Reactive hypoglycemia
    - Alimentary
    - "Pre-diabetes"
    - Endocrine
    - Idiopathic
- Factitious
    - Surreptitious insulin administration
    - Surreptitious sulfonylurea administration
    - Factitious hypoglycemia is extremely difficult to discern. If the patient uses insulin, there may be a low level of C-peptide, but if a sulfonylureas is being used, then insulin and C-peptide may be elevated. In this case look for the presence of insulin antibodies and sulfonylureas.
- Postprandial hypoglycemia due to bariatric surgery
- Hyperinsulinemia
    - An accurate diagnosis of organic hyperinsulinemia can be established in most cases by a process of exclusion. The diagnosis can usually be made before extensive exploration of neoplastic causes.
- Autoimmunity
    - Syndromes of autoimmunity may lead to hypoglycemia. Antireceptor antibodies usually occur in the presence of other autoimmune disease,

mimicking the effect of insulin and reducing insulin clearance. Insulin levels may be normal or high, but C-peptide levels are low because islet cells are suppressed.

- Reactive hypoglycemia
    - Autoimmune hypoglycemic disease syndrome usually occurs in the presence of other autoimmune disorders (e.g., Graves' disease, rheumatoid arthritis, lupus) and commonly produces reactive hypoglycemia from prolongation of the half-life of circulating insulin. This is also an important mechanism in late dumping syndrome. Insulin levels are generally extremely elevated, which may result from interference by antibodies with the particular insulin assay. C-peptide levels are usually low.
- Neoplasms
    - In the case of large mesenchymal neoplasms or sarcomas, the offending agent may be IGF-2; neither the size of the tumor nor the glucose metabolized by the tumor causes hyperglycemia; however, there is increased disposal of glucose by the liver mimicking the actions of insulin.
- Counter-regulatory hormone deficiency
    - Hypoglycemia resulting from conditions in which there is failure of gluconeogenesis or hormonal counter-regulations for (e.g. Addison's disease), hypopituitarism usually can be recognized clinically.

Non–Islet Cell Neoplasms Associated With Hypoglycemia

- Mesenchymal
    - Mesothelioma
    - Fibrosarcoma
    - Rhabdomyosarcoma
    - Leiomyosarcoma
    - Hemangiopericytoma
- Carcinoma
    - Hepatic: hepatoma, biliary carcinoma
    - Adrenocortical carcinoma
    - Genitourinary: hypernephroma, Wilms' tumor of the prostate
    - Reproductive: cervical or breast carcinoma
- Neurologic/neuroendocrine
    - Pheochromocytoma
    - Carcinoid
    - Neurofibroma
- Hematologic
    - Leukemia
    - Lymphoma
    - Myeloma

The Next Step

Hormones, Peptides, and Enzymes

- Insulin
- IGF-2
- C-peptide
- Glucagon-like peptide type 1 (GLP-1) and GIP
- Sulfonylurea
- ACTH
- GH
- Insulin antibodies
- Liver enzymes

ICD-10 CODE: Hypoglycemia E16.2
Diabetic E10.649 or E11.649
Due to insulin E16.0
Reactive E16.1

ICD-10 CODE: Hyperinsulinemia E16.1

ICD-10 CODE: Dumping Syndrome
Nonsurgical K30
Postgastrectomy K91.1

ICD-10 CODE: Complications of Drug Injection or Therapy T88.8XXA

ICD-10 CODE: Complication of Surgical Procedure T81.9XXA

(See Table 1-1 for primary tumor sites and common metastatic tumor sites)
(See Hypoglycemia/Insulinoma Screening Test [Chapter 5] for specific tests and CPT codes [Chapter 4])

DERMOPATHY

When dermopathy occurs with glucagonoma syndrome it is also known by the acronym 4D, which stands for dermatosis, diarrhea, deep vein thrombosis (DVT), and depression. Pellagra- like eruptions occur in carcinoid as a result of niacin deficiency, and increased pigmentation occurs with MSH overproduction.

WHAT TO LOOK FOR

Distinguishing Signs and Symptoms

- Characteristic NME rash (82%)
- Pellagra rash forming a necklace and forearm pigmentation with the appearance of tiling
- Increased pigmentation in sun-exposed areas with overproduction of MSH
- Painful glossitis, angular stomatitis
- Normochromic normocytic anemia (61%)
- Weight loss (90%)
- Mild diabetes mellitus (80%)
- Hypoaminoacidemia
- Deep Vein Thrombosis (DVT) (>50%)
- Depression (50%)

THE NEXT STEP

Hormones, Peptides, and Amino Acids

- Glucagon
- Plasma amino acids (tryptophan)
- α-MSH
- Serotonin
- 5-HIAA (plasma)
- Niacin

ICD-10 CODE: Glucagonoma —For Glucagonoma Rash
   Malignant
      Pancreas C25.4
      Unspecified site C25.9
      Specified site–see Neoplasm by site, malignant
   Benign
      Specified site–see Neoplasm by site, benign
      Unspecified site D13.7
   Uncertain behavior, neoplasm of pancreas D37.8
   Islets of Langerhans D13.7

ICD-10 CODE: Pellagra E52

(See Table 1-1 for primary tumor sites and common metastatic tumor sites)
(See Glucagon [Chapter 4] and Serotonin [Chapter 4] for specific tests and CPT codes)

DUMPING SYNDROME

Postgastrectomy dumping syndrome occurs in as many as 25% of patients undergoing ablative or bypass surgery on the pylorus. Approximately 5% of patients have debilitating dumping syndrome following major gastric resections. There may be varying degrees of this pathophysiologic state. Ingestion of cold or carbohydrate-rich foods may precipitate early dumping with cardiovascular (tachycardia and shock-like symptoms) and gastrointestinal components (explosive diarrhea and cramping). Classically, patients with dumping syndrome do not have symptoms with every meal; therefore, they commonly use medication to control this syndrome only when they know that they are going to ingest foods that will provoke an attack. Late dumping is characterized by hypoglycemic events. These features can be explained by insulin-induced hypoglycemia. Alterations in gut peptide levels have been implicated in both early and late dumping syndromes. PP, glucagon, insulin, and motilin have been implicated in the pathogenesis of dumping syndrome.

WHAT TO LOOK FOR

Distinguishing Signs and Symptoms Early Dumping Syndrome

Early dumping is caused by rapid shifts of water and electrolytes into the duodenum and proximal small bowel lumen in response to the introduction of hyperosmolar chyme into these regions. Fluid shifts into the gut lumen produce intravascular volume reduction, subsequent hemoconcentration, and an adrenergic shock-like response, producing the following symptoms:
- Diaphoresis
- Syncope
- Tachycardia
- Hypotension
- Borborygmus
- Explosive diarrhea

Late Dumping Syndrome

- Tremors
- Diaphoresis
- Syncope
- Mental confusion

THE NEXT STEP

Carbohydrate Test

Use a high-carbohydrate test meal to provoke dumping syndrome in a controlled clinical environment. This test meal contains 750 kcal, 21g protein, 30 g fat, and 99 g of carbohydrate (i.e., 2 eggs, 2 strips of bacon, a cup of decaffeinated coffee, 2 pieces of toast, 1 scoop of ice cream, and 1 ounce of chocolate syrup). The meal must be consumed within 10 minutes. Patients with dumping syndrome usually respond with significant rises in PP, insulin, and glucagon levels within 45 minutes of ingestion of this meal. Increases in motilin levels are usually seen 120 to 180 minutes after ingestion of a provocative meal.

Hormones and Peptides

- Insulin
- PP (pancreatic polypeptide)
- Glucagon
- GIP
- GLP-1, Total
- Motilin

Octreotide Suppression Test

Octreotide acetate administration at low doses (100 µg 1 hour before meals) has been effectively used to control the symptoms of early dumping but is less efficacious in the control of late dumping. It can however, be used as a test of hormone and symptom responsiveness. Use of octreotide in patients with late dumping syndrome can be associated with worsening of hypoglycemia and should be done only in a controlled clinical environment.

ICD-10 CODE: Dumping Syndrome
Nonsurgical K31.89
Postgastrectomy K91.1

(See Table 1-1 for primary tumor sites and common metastatic tumor sites)
(See further test instructions and CPT codes for specific hormone and peptide measurements [Chapter 4], Provocative Test for Dumping Syndrome [Chapter 6])

PITUITARY AND HYPOTHALAMIC DISORDERS

Diseases of the hypothalamus and pituitary and ectopic production of hypothalamic hormones produce syndromes of hormone excess or deficiency. Non-secreting pituitary tumors may present with only signs and symptoms of mass effect on adjacent structures (i.e., optic chiasm, cranial nerves 3 and 4 and branches thereof, cranial nerves 5 and 6 as they traverse the cavernous sinus, and the sphenoid sinus) if enough normal pituitary remains to prevent hypopituitarism.

Diseases of Hormonal Excess

- Hyperprolactinemia
- Acromegaly and gigantism
- Cushing's syndrome
- Other pituitary hypersecretion syndromes
    - TSHomas
    - Gonadotropin- or human glycoprotein alpha subunit– (α-GSU) secreting pituitary adenomas

HYPERPROLACTINEMIA

The clinical effects of prolactin excess vary according to the time of onset of the disease.

WHAT TO LOOK FOR

Distinguishing Signs and Symptoms Children

- Hypogonadism with pubertal delay or arrest
- Absent pubertal growth spurt due to hypogonadism

Women

- Hypogonadism
    - Infertility
    - Oligorrhea/amenorrhea
- Galactorrhea
- Hirsutism due to stimulation of adrenal androgen

ICD-10 CODE: Amenorrhea N91.2
Ovarian dysfunction E28.9
Hyperhormonal E28.8

ICD-10 CODE: Galactorrhea
In pregnancy O92.6
Not associated with childbirth N64.3

ICD-10 CODE: Hirsutism L68.0

ICD-10 CODE: Hypogonadism
Ovarian E28.39
Testicular E29.1

ICD-10 CODE: Hyperprolactinemia E22.1

ICD-10 CODE: MEN-1 Syndrome E31.21

ICD-10 CODE: Oligomenorrhea N91.3-N91.5

(See MEN Syndrome Screen [Chapter 5] and Pituitary and Hypothalamic Disorders Tests [Chapter 6] for specific tests and CPT codes)

ACROMEGALY AND GIGANTISM

Growth hormone is secreted by the anterior pituitary. Its release is controlled by GH-RH and somatostatin. GH is also known as somatotropin and is in the family of compounds known as somatomammotropins, which includes prolactin and human placental lactogen. GH stimulates production of RNA, resulting in increased anabolism. GH levels are elevated in persons with pituitary gigantism and in those with acromegaly that is characterized by growth after the epiphyses have closed resulting in abnormal bone growth of face, hands, and feet. GH levels are decreased in persons with dwarfism. Patients taking GH therapy frequently develop GH antibodies, which act to negate the biologic effect of the medication.

The clinical effects of GH excess vary according to the time of onset of the disease. Relative frequency of symptoms in acromegaly is shown in **Table 3-4**.

Table 3-4. The Relative Frequency of Symptoms in Acromegaly

Clinical Features	Percentage
Enlargement of extremities	99
Facial coarsening	97
Visceromegaly	92
Necessity to increase shoe size	88
Necessity to increase ring size	87
Sella enlargement	83
Acroparesthesias	82
Arthralgia	80
Hyperhidrosis, seborrhea	78
Arthrosis	76
Teeth separation	75
Frontal bossing	72
Oily skin	70
Malocclusion and overbite	65
Prognathism	65
Headache	62
Sleep apnea	52
High blood pressure	42
Impaired glucose tolerance	40
Skin tags	38
Goiter	38
Menstrual abnormalities	36
Asthenia	35
Sexual disturbances	34
Carpal tunnel syndrome	28
Overt diabetes	28
Visual field defects	27
Galactorrhea	4
Cranial nerve palsies	3

WHAT TO LOOK FOR

Distinguishing Signs and Symptoms

The somatic changes in children include the following:
- Increase in growth velocity
- Gigantism

The changes in adults and children include the following:
- Enlargement of the extremities (hands, feet, nose, mandible, and supraorbital ridges) compelling patients to seek large gloves, shoes, and rings
- Development of thick skin which is moist, oily, and seborrheic with an increase in sebaceous cysts and skin tags
- Acanthosis nigricans and hypertrichosis
- Widely spaced teeth
- Visceromegaly of the tongue, liver, thyroid, and salivary glands
- Overgrowth of bone and cartilage causing degenerative changes in spine, hips, and knees
- Arthralgia and paresthesias
- Nerve entrapments, particularly of the median nerve but also ulnar and peroneal

Diagnosis of Acromegaly

The basal level of GH and IGF-1 is usually sufficient to make the diagnosis. However, in 15% to 25% of cases, the levels of GH are less than 10 ng/mL and the IGF-1 level may be normal. In these instances it is important to show nonsuppressibility of GH to an oral glucose tolerance test (or a somatostatin inhibition or bromocryptine suppression test). Levels of other pituitary hormones such as prolactin and the α subunit of gonadotropins are also often elevated; measure these as well as thyroid-stimulating hormone (TSH). If ordering a glucose tolerance test, measure GH in addition to glucose, because the criterion for diagnosis of acromegaly is based on suppression of GH and insulin as well as lipids.

THE NEXT STEP

Imaging of the sella turcica will show a tumor. In the absence of a tumor and the suggestion of hyperplasia, evaluate for a hypothalamic hamartoma or ectopic production of GH-RH. If the GH-RH level is greater than 300 pg/mL, CT and MRI of the pancreas, gastroduodenal area, thymus, and lungs should facilitate a diagnosis.

Because these NETs express somatostatin receptors, OctreoScan will often reveal their location. In about 20% of patients a pituitary tumor will coexist with MEN-1 syndrome; thus it is important to also measure ionized calcium and PTH.

The radiologic study of bones will show thickening of the skull, enlargement of the frontal and maxillary sinuses, prognathism, tufting of the phalanges, and cysts in carpal and tarsal bones. Soft tissue enlargement can be seen, particularly with heel pad thickness. In patients over 50 years old, colonic polyps may become carcinomas, particularly in people with skin tags. For these patients, routine sequential colonoscopy is recommended. The flow diagram presented in **Figure 3-3** suggests the diagnostic workup.

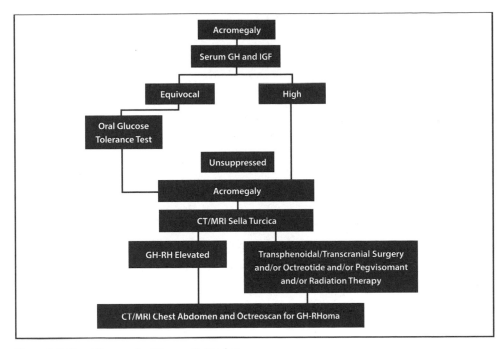

Figure 3-3. Flow Diagram for Diagnostic Workup

Hormones and Peptides

- GH
- IGF-1
- Prolactin
- TSH
- GH-RH if no tumor visualized or pituitary hyperplasia on MRI
- PTH

Measure the following:
- GH and IGF-1
- Oral glucose tolerance test; also measure GH, insulin, and lipids
- Somatostatin inhibition test
- Bromocryptine suppression test
- Prolactin
- TSH
- Ionized calcium
- PTH

ICD-10 CODE: Acromegaly E22.0

ICD-10 CODE: Gigantism E22.0

ICD-10 CODE: MEN-1 Syndrome E31.21

(See Growth Hormone [HGH, Somatotropin] [Chapter 4] and Thyroid Stimulating Hormone [TSH, Thyrotropin] [Chapter 4] for specific tests and CPT codes)

CUSHING'S SYNDROME

In Cushing's disease, oversecretion of pituitary ACTH induces bilateral adrenal hyperplasia. This results in excess production of cortisol, adrenal androgens, and 11-deoxycorticosterone. Cushing's disease, a subset of Cushing's syndrome, is due to a pituitary corticotroph adenoma and results in a partial resistance to the suppression of ACTH by cortisol so that secretion is unrestrained. In contrast, causes of Cushing's syndrome may include the following:

- Adrenal adenoma or carcinoma arise spontaneously. ACTH levels are undetectable.
- Nonpituitary (ectopic) tumors produce ACTH. They most frequently originate in the thorax and are highly aggressive small cell carcinomas of the lung or slow-growing bronchial or thymic carcinoid tumors. Some produce corticotropin-releasing hormone (CRH) instead, which stimulates pituitary ACTH secretion and can therefore mimic a pituitary tumor.
- Other causes include carcinoid tumors of the gastric, pancreatic, and intestinal organs; pheochromocytomas, and MCT.

The hallmark of Cushing's syndrome is that ACTH levels are partially resistant to suppression with dexamethasone, even at very high doses.

WHAT TO LOOK FOR

Distinguishing Signs and Symptoms

The clinical features of common varieties of Cushing's disease include or are related to the following:

- Fat and protein metabolism
- Centripetal weight gain
- Development of the buffalo hump
- Supraclavicular fat pads
- Plethoric moon face
- Thin skin
- Little accumulation of subcutaneous fat over the dorsum of the hand and shin
- Purple striae, often greater than 1 cm wide, usually located over the abdomen but not in traditional stretch areas
- Slow healing of minor wounds
- Muscle wasting in the proximal lower limbs leading to inability to rise from a chair and weakness
- Bone wasting resulting in generalized osteoporosis
- Kyphosis and loss of height
- Elevated blood pressure
- Fluid accumulation leading to congestive heart failure
- Evidence of androgen excess with hirsutism in women
- Clitoromegaly
- Coarsening of the skin
- Hoarse voice due to the androgen excess, particularly true in adrenocortical carcinomas
- Psychic disturbances
- Anxiety
- Emotional lability
- Depression
- Unwarranted euphoria with sleep disturbances

The nonpituitary or ectopic ACTH syndrome is often diagnosed because of its rapid onset and progress. Classically the condition is dominated by the following characteristics:
- Profound muscle wasting
- Electrolyte disturbances
- Severe hypokalemia
- Overproduction of mineralocorticoids
- Impaired insulin secretion resulting in diabetes
- Striking pigmentation due to the structural homology of ACTH and MSH

This pigmentation contrasts with the absence of pigmentation in classic Cushing's disease and adrenal tumors, in which ACTH is suppressed.

The Next Step

Increased urinary cortisol and plasma cortisol suggest Cushing's disease. A suppressed ACTH level indicates the presence of an adrenal tumor. Mildly elevated ACTH directs attention to the pituitary. Markedly elevated ACTH suggests a small cell carcinoma of the lung or an ectopic carcinoid type of tumor.

Hormones and Peptides

- ACTH
- Cortisol
- Adrenal
- Androgens
- 11-Deoxycorticosterone
- MSH (Alpha- or Beta- and Gamma-Melanocyte Stimulating Hormone)

First-Line Screening

1. Measure plasma ACTH, cortisol, and 24-hour urinary free cortisol excretion.
2. Repeat at least three 24-hour urinary free cortisol collections if high clinical suspicion exists. One or more collections may be normal due to "cyclic Cushing's disease," and in preclinical Cushing's syndrome, the urinary free cortisol may be normal.
3. Perform low-dose dexamethasone suppression test (DST) either overnight (1 mg between 11:00 PM and 12:00 AM) or 0.5 mg every 6 hours for 48 hours. N–1 suppression is to less than 1.8 µg/dL (50 nmol/L).
4. Measure circadian rhythm of cortisol by obtaining serum Cortisol levels at 8:00 to 9:30 AM, 4:30 to 6:00 PM, and 11:00 PM to 12:00 AM. For the latter measurement, patient should be asleep as an inpatient after 48 hours (only if not acutely ill); if patient is not in the hospital, or is acutely ill, obtain a salivary cortisol level.

(See Pituitary and Hypothalamic Tests [Chapter 6] for more details on ACTH and cortisol testing)

Second-Line Screening

1. Measure circadian rhythm of cortisol, as above.
2. Perform low-dose DST 0.5 mg for 48 hours with measurement of 24-hour urinary free cortisol on the second day. Excretion of less than 10 µg/24 hours (27 nmol/L) is normal.
3. Perform low-dose DST (0.5 mg every 6 hours for 48 hours) followed by CRH stimulation (100 µg or 1 µg/kg of intravenous ovine CRH). A cortisol response greater than 1.4 µg/dL at 15 minutes is consistent with Cushing's disease.

(See Pituitary and Hypothalamic Tests [Chapter 5] for more details on cortisol testing, low-dose DST, and low-dose DST with CRH stimulation)

What You Need to Know if Cushing's Syndrome Is Confirmed

1. If ACTH is easily detectable (>20 pg/mL, or 4 pmol/L) focus on the pituitary with MRI of the sella turcica. This test is positive in 50% to 60% of cases of proven pituitary Cushing's disease.

2. If ACTH level is less than 20 pg/mL, prove that it is suppressed with a CRH test. Administer CRH 1 µg/kg or 100 µg/1 kg (but *not* dexamethasone) as described previously, and measure ACTH in addition to cortisol at 15, 30, and 45 minutes after CRH. An increase of greater than 50% in ACTH supports a pituitary tumor; ectopic ACTH-secreting tumors generally (but not invariably) do not respond to CRH. Those that do are carcinoids tumors of bronchus, thymus, or pancreas; islet cell tumors; MCTs, or pheochromocytomas, rather than the more common small cell carcinomas of the lung.

3. Perform high-dose DST. High doses of glucocorticoids partially suppress ACTH secretion from 80% to 90% of corticotroph adenomas, whereas ectopic tumors usually resist negative feedback inhibition. However, as discussed previously, some benign NETs may be sensitive to feedback inhibition of ACTH, similar to pituitary tumors. In adrenal-based Cushing's syndrome, plasma cortisol is not suppressed after high-dose DST because cortisol secretion is autonomous and pituitary ACTH secretion is already suppressed. As with the low-dose DST, there are several versions of the high-dose DST, including the standard 2-day oral high dose (2 mg every 6 hours for 48 hours), the 8-mg overnight oral, the intravenous 4 mg, and the ultra-high-dose (8 mg every 6 hours) tests. Plasma and/or urinary cortisol levels are evaluated before, during, and/or after DST. Suppression of plasma cortisol to 50% of baseline provides a specificity of up to 80%.

4. Perform inferior petrosal sinus sampling. If the above tests point to an ACTH-dependent process but no adenoma is evident on MRI, the next step should be bilateral inferior petrosal sinus sampling. An experienced radiologist catheterizes both inferior petrosal sinuses, and samples for ACTH are obtained simultaneously from both the sinuses and a peripheral vein before and at 3, 5, and 10 minutes after intravenous administration of ovine CRH (1 µg/kg or 100 µg/1 kg). An inferior petrosal sinus–to–peripheral ACTH ratio greater than 2.0 at baseline or after CRH administration is consistent with Cushing's disease. Lower ratios suggest an ectopic ACTH-secreting tumor. A side-to-side ratio of 1.4 or greater may provide direction to neurosurgeons performing transsphenoidal hypophysectomy when no tumor is evident on MRI.

In Search of Occult Ectopic ACTH-Secreting Tumors

If bilateral inferior petrosal sinus sampling confirms the lack of a pituitary ACTH gradient, perform CT and/or MRI of the neck, thorax, and abdomen, because most nonpituitary ACTH-secreting tumors are NETs, as noted previously. Additionally, perform MRI of the chest, because this imaging procedure may uncover (central) bronchial carcinoids missed by CT. Somatostatin analog scintigraphy with ^{111}In-pentetreotide (OctreoScan) may identify a few occult ACTH-secreting tumors with somatostatin receptors that were not clearly identified by CT or MRI imaging. Positron emission tomography scanning may also prove helpful in the search for occult ACTH-secreting tumors.

Other procedures that have been used to discriminate between pituitary-dependent and ectopic ACTH syndromes include desmopressin with or without CRH; the GH secretogogues hexarelin and ghrelin, which stimulate ACTH in patients with pituitary adenomas, but not in normals, and the opiate agonist loperamide, which suppresses normals, but not patients with Cushing's disease. None of these research procedures can be recommended for standard clinical practice as of yet.

ICD-10 CODE: Cushing's Syndrome/Cushing's Disease E24.0-E24.9

(See [Chapter 4] for specific tests and CPT codes)

Other Pituitary Hypersecretion Syndromes

TSH-Secreting Pituitary Adenomas (TSHoma)

Thyroid-stimulating hormone is a glycoprotein produced in the pituitary consisting of two subunits: α and β. The α subunit is identical or similar to that of follicle-stimulating hormone (FSH), luteinizing hormone (LH), and chorionic gonadotropin. The β subunit is specific to TSH. The secretion of TSH is controlled by release of thyrotropin-releasing hormone (TRH) from the hypothalamus. TSH stimulates all metabolic and cellular processes involved in synthesis and secretion of thyroid hormones. TSH also stimulates intermediary metabolism and thyroid growth. TSH initiates release of thyroxine and triiodothyronine from thyroglobulin. TSH is increased in almost all cases of primary hypothyroidism and decreased in most cases of hyperthyroidism; TSH thyrotoxicosis is one exception. TSH secretion is increased by estrogens and suppressed by androgens and corticosteroids.

Thyrotropin-releasing hormone is a tripeptide produced primarily by the hypothalamus. TRH is produced from a prohormone that contains multiple copies of the TRH molecule. Several TRH entities can be released from one precursor. TRH has a stimulatory effect on the pituitary, causing it to release TSH. TRH secretion is controlled by hormones via a negative feedback system. Binding of TRH to its receptor causes a rise in calcium, which initiates TSH secretion. It also stimulates adenyl cyclase in the pituitary. Additionally, TRH stimulates secretion of prolactin, GH in acromegaly, and ACTH in Cushing's and Nelson's syndromes. Levels of TRH are undetectable or very low in patients with hyperthyroidism and hypothalamic hypothyroidism. Levels are elevated in patients with primary and pituitary hypothyroidism.

What to Look For

Distinguishing Signs and Symptoms

- Approximately 300 cases have been reported in the last 35 years. Previously, TSHomas were not found until they had grown to macroadenoma size (>10 mm); more recently, some of these tumors have been discovered at the microadenoma size as a result of the 100-fold increase in sensitivity in TSH assays.
- When pituitary adenomas secrete TSH, they are autonomous and refractory to the negative feedback of thyroid hormones (i.e., inappropriate TSH secretion) and can produce hyperthyroidism. Thus, the key finding is detectable serum TSH levels in the presence of elevated free triiodothyronine (T4) and free thyroxine (T3) concentrations. TSH concentrations may be elevated or normal.
- Earlier diagnosis and treatment directed at the pituitary, as opposed to the thyroid, may prevent the loss of visual field caused by impingement on the optic chiasm and hypopituitarism that occur as the tumors enlarge, and furthermore may improve the rate of neurosurgical cure.
- TSHomas present with signs and symptoms of hyperthyroidism including goiter, and 25% of these tumors show mixed pituitary hormone secretion, usually GH or prolactin, thus patients should be evaluated for galactorrhea/amenorrhea and acromegaly.

THE NEXT STEP

Hormones and Peptides

- TRH
- TSH
- Free T4 and free T3
- Prolactin
- GH and IGF-1
- α-GSU
- LH, FSH
- Testosterone, sex hormone–binding globulin, or estradiol
- Cortisol and ACTH

Dynamic testing may be required to uncover hypocortisolism. See Pituitary and Hypothalamic Disorders, discussed earlier in this chapter.

Dynamic Suppression Testing

- T3 suppression test (75–100 µg/d orally in divided doses for 8–10 days). Inhibition of TSH secretion after T3 suppression test has never been recorded in patients with TSHoma. However, this test is strictly contraindicated in elderly patients or in those with coronary heart disease.
- TRH suppression test. Widely used to investigate the presence of a TSHoma. The TRH test is available from ISI and must be collected with use of special TRH Preservative tube to prevent degradation of the molecule. [See Chapter 4 for special collection instructions.] After intravenous administration of 200 microgram TRH, TSH andα-GSU levels generally do not increase in patients with TSHoma.
- Somatostatin suppression test. Administration of somatostatin or its analogs (octreotide and lanreotide) reduces TSH levels in most cases and may predict the efficacy of long-term treatment, but it is not considered diagnostic for TSHoma.

Imaging Studies and Localization of the Tumor

Nuclear MRI is preferred for imaging other tumors of the sella turcica, such as TSHomas. CT may be used as an alternative to MRI in patients with contraindication (e.g., pacemaker, claustrophobia).

GONADOTROPIN OR α-GSU–SECRETING PITUITARY ADENOMAS

Many pituitary adenomas stain positively for either LH or FSH or for their α-glycoprotein subunit (and also that of TSH and human chorionic gonadotropin); few patients have elevated gonadotropin levels. Gonadotropinomas (or α-GSUomas) generally present as macroadenomas with visual field loss, headaches, or hypopituitarism including infertility, early menopause, or male hypogonadism.

In general, elevations of both LH and FSH imply primary hypogonadism rather than gonadotropinoma. Because α-GSU is frequently secreted in mixed or "silent" pituitary adenomas, its concentration should be measured as part of the evaluation of any pituitary adenoma.

ICD-10 CODE: Pituitary Syndrome E22.0

ICD-10 CODE: Other/Unspecified Anterior Pituitary Hyperfunction E22.9

ICD-10 CODE: Thyrotoxicosis of Other Specified Origin Without Mention of Crisis or Storm E05.40

ICD-10 CODE: Thyrotoxicosis of Other Specified Origin With Mention of Crisis or Storm E05.81

ICD-10 CODES for Pituitary Neoplasm

Site	Malignant	Benign	Uncertain Behavior	Unspecified
Pituitary gland	C75.1	D35.2	D44.3	D49.7

(See [Chapter 4] for specific tests and CPT codes)

PITUITARY HORMONE INSUFFICIENCY (CHILDHOOD)

Multiple childhood tumors can affect pituitary function, including craniopharyngioma, germinoma, hamartoma, low-grade astrocytoma, Langerhans' cell histiocytosis, and dermoid and epidermoid tumors. These generally compress the hypothalamus or, in the case of craniopharyngioma and germinoma, the pituitary stalk. Benign pituitary adenomas frequently affect the anterior pituitary. Common posterior pituitary lesions include astrocytoma and Langerhans' cell histiocytosis.

WHAT TO LOOK FOR

Distinguishing Signs and Symptoms

- Raised intracranial pressure caused by expansion of tumor with obstruction of the cerebrospinal fluid (CSF), causing headaches, vomiting, and papilledema.
- Cranial nerve palsies, visual field defects, and hypothalamo-hypophyseal dysfunction (one third of cases as the initial presentation).
- Hyposecretion (and occasionally hypersecretion) of pituitary hormones. These are usually easy to recognize.
- Hypothalamo-pituitary syndromes, characterized by variable endocrine disturbances, occur in association with hypothalamic dysfunction. (The hypothalamus is important for the control of many basic cerebral functions, such as appetite, emotion, and temperature homeostasis.)
- Craniopharyngioma and peripituitary lesions with suprasellar extension may cause visual difficulties due to the compression of the optic nerves and/or chiasm.
- Hypopituitarism. Usually, hormone loss is sequential, beginning with loss of GH secretion, followed by gonadotropins, TSH, and ACTH. In children, in contrast to adults, the loss of GH secretion is usually more obvious with growth failure and possibly hypoglycemia.
- Central precocious puberty, defined as signs of puberty (breast development in girls, and increase in testicular volume in boys) occurring under the age of 8 years in a girl and 8.5 years in a boy. These symptoms are gonadotropin-dependent and therefore are ameliorated by long-acting gonadotropin-releasing hormone agonists, which downregulate the pituitary gonadotropin-releasing hormone receptors.
- Hypothalamopituitary tumors in the peripubertal age range may present as failure to enter puberty or arrested pubertal development and consequent blunted or even absent growth spurt.

If onset of gonadotropin-releasing hormone insufficiency occurs during fetal development (i.e., congenital), the male genitalia will be abnormal, with micropenis and bilateral small undescended testes due to failure of testosterone secretion in utero. Under these circumstances, perform MRI of the olfactory bulbs/grooves to seek evidence of Kallmann's syndrome.

ICD-10 CODE: Hypopituitarism E23.0
Hormone therapy E23.1
Hypophysectomy E89.3
Radiotherapy E89.3
Postablative E89.3
Postpartum hemorrhage E23.0

(See [Chapter 4] for specific tests and CPT codes)

DIABETES INSIPIDUS (ADULTHOOD)

Vasopressin is derived from the supraoptic and periventricular nuclei of the hypothalamus and is released from the nerve endings in the neurohypophysis (i.e.,posterior pituitary). Before overt diabetes insipidus occurs, 85% to 90% of vasopressin secretion must be lost. New-onset diabetes insipidus should raise suspicion of a tumor, although 50% of acquired cases have an autoimmune etiology. Tumors may be occult for many years; thus, patients often require serial neuroimaging to reveal the diagnosis.

CAUSES

Hypothalamic (Central) Diabetes Insipidus (HDI)

- Congenital
    - Genetic: Wolfram syndrome or diabetes insipidus, diabetes mellitus, optic atrophy, and deafness (DIDMOAD)
    - Developmental syndromes: septo-optic dysplasia, Lawrence-Moon-Biedel syndrome
- Idiopathic
- Acquired
    - Trauma
    - Neurosurgical injury (transcranial, transsphenoidal)
- Tumor
    - Craniopharyngioma, pinealoma, germinoma, metastases, pituitary macroadenoma (unusual cause as it is a hypothalamic disease)
- Inflammatory
    - Granulomas
    - Sarcoid
    - Tuberculous meningitis
    - Langerhans' cell histiocytosis
    - Meningitis, encephalitis
- Infundibuloneurohypophysitis
- Autoimmune
    - Anti-vasopressin neuron antibodies
- Vascular
    - Aneurysm
    - Infarction: Sheehan's syndrome, sickle cell disease
- Pregnancy (associated with vasopressinase)

Nephrogenic Diabetes Insipidus (NDI)

- Genetic
    - X-linked recessive (V2-R defect)
    - Autosomal recessive (AQP2 defect)
    - Autosomal dominant (AQP2 defect)
- Idiopathic
- Chronic renal disease (e.g., polycystic kidneys)
- Metabolic disease
    - Hypercalcemia
    - Hypokalemia
- Drug induced
    - Lithium

- - Demeclocycline
- - Platinum-based antineoplastic drugs
- Osmotic diuretics
  - - Glucose
  - - Mannitol
  - - Urea (post–obstructive uropathy)
- Systemic disorders
  - - Amyloidosis
  - - Myelomatosis
- Pregnancy

Dipsogenic Diabetes Insipidus (DDI)

- Compulsive water drinking associated with psychologic disorders (i.e., psychogenic polydypsia)
- Drug induced

Structural/Organic Hypothalamic Disease

- Tumors involving hypothalamus
- Head injury

Granulomatous Diseases

- Sarcoid
- Tuberculous meningitis
- Langerhans' cell histiocytosis

WHAT TO LOOK FOR

Distinguishing Signs and Symptoms

- Thirst
- Polydipsia
- Polyuria

Exclude the following conditions:
- Hyperglycemia
- Hypokalemia
- Hypercalcemia
- Renal insufficiency

Measure the following values:
- 24-hour urine volume (abnormal is >40 mL/kg/24 hours)
- Serum sodium (This will generally be maintained in the high-normal range in HDI patients, and alternatively, be in the low-normal range in DDI patients.)
- Glucose
- Blood urea nitrogen (BUN)
- Serum and urine osmolality
- Plasma vasopressin

THE NEXT STEP

Request water deprivation/desmopressin test to determine whether HDI, NDI, or DDI.
- HDI: urine osmolality is less than 300 mOsm/kg accompanied by plasma osmolality greater than 290 mOsm/kg after dehydration; urine osmolality should rise above 750 mOsm/kg after desmopressin acetate (DDAVP)
- NDI: failure to increase urine osmolality above 300 mOsm/kg after dehydration, with no response to DDAVP
- DDI: appropriate urine concentration during dehydration without significant rise in plasma osmolality

If HDI is diagnosed, the next step should be imaging of the hypothalamus/perisellar region with MRI to exclude possible tumors. HDI frequently is associated with loss of the normal posterior pituitary bright spot on T1-weighted MRI, which correlates with posterior pituitary vasopressin content.

For more information go to: http://www.endotext.com/neuroendo/neuroendo11a/neuroendoframe11a.htm (Children) http://www.endotext.com/neuroendo/neuroendo2/neuroendoframe2.htm (Diabetes Insipidus and Syndrome of Inappropriate Antidiuretic Hormone [SIADH])

ICD-10 CODE: Diabetes Insipidus E23.2

ICD-10 CODE: Nephrogenic Diabetes Insipidus N25.1

ICD-10 CODE: Pituitary Diabetes Insipidus E23.2

ICD-10 CODE: Vasopressin-Resistant Diabetes Insipidus N25.1

(See [Chapter 4] for specific tests and CPT codes)

HYPONATREMIA AND SYNDROME OF INAPPROPRIATE ANTIDIURETIC HORMONE (SIADH)

Hyponatremia (serum sodium level <135 mEq/L) and hypo-osmolality are the most common fluid and electrolyte disorders in hospitalized patients with hyponatremia and syndrome of inappropriate antidiuretic hormone (SIADH). Hyponatremia is important clinically because severe hypo-osmolality (serum sodium level <120 mEq/L) is associated with substantial morbidity and mortality. Excessively rapid correction of hyponatremia can itself cause severe neurologic morbidity and mortality due to osmotic demyelinization (i.e., central pontine demyelinization).

WHAT TO LOOK FOR

Distinguishing Signs and Symptoms

- Lethargy
- Anorexia
- Headache
- Nausea
- Vomiting
- Muscle cramps
- Disorientation
- Seizure
- Coma
- Death

Criteria for Diagnosis of Hyponatremia Due to SIADH

- Hyponatremia with appropriately low plasma osmolality (<280 mOsm/kg)
- Urine osmolality greater than 100 mOsm/kg (i.e., less than maximally dilute) at a time when the plasma is hypo-osmolar
- Renal (urine) sodium excretion greater than 30 mM/L
- Absence of hypotension, hypovolemia, and edema-forming states
- Normal cardiac, renal, pituitary, thyroid, and adrenal function

Differential Diagnosis

Plasma osmolality can be calculated as (mOsm/kg H3O) = 2x [Na] (mEq/L) + glucose (mg/dL)/18 + BUN (mg/dL)/2.8 and is accurate under usual conditions but can be misleading under the following conditions:

- Pseudohyponatremia, which is due to gross hyperlipidemia (triglycerides or cholesterol) or serum proteins
- Isotonic or hypertonic hyponatremia, which is due to high concentrations of other solutes (e.g., glucose, mannitol, alcohols/ethylene glycol, radiocontrast dyes, urea) Hypotonic hyponatremia is best determined by directly measuring plasma osmolality.

If direct and calculated measurements agree, then calculated osmolality can be used subsequently.

Measure the following levels:
- Plasma osmolality
- Serum sodium
- Glucose
- BUN
- Ethanol, methanol, etc. (depending on the situation)
- Urine osmolality
- Urine sodium
- Serum uric acid

Causes of Hypotonic Hyponatremia

- Sodium depletion
  - Renal loss
  - Diuretics
  - Salt-wasting nephropathy
  - Central salt wasting
- Extrarenal loss
  - GI losses (vomiting, diarrhea)
  - Sweating
  - Hemorrhage
- Hypoadrenalism (renal losses if primary, decreased free water excretion in primary or secondary)
- Reduced renal free water clearance
  - Hypovolemia
  - Cardiac failure
  - Nephrotic syndrome
  - Hypothyroidism
  - Renal failure
  - Ascites
  - Hypoalbuminemia
  - Sepsis and vascular leak syndromes
  - Fluid sequestration
- Excess water intake
  - DDI at times when water intake exceeds renal clearance
  - Sodium-free, hyposomolar irrigant solutions
  - Dilute infant feeding formula
  - SIADH

Causes of Drug-Induced Hyponatremia

- Saline depletion: diuretics, spironolactone, thiazides, loop diuretics plus angiotensin-converting enzyme (ACE) inhibitors, angiotensin receptor blockers

Causes of Vasopressin-Like Activity

- DDAVP
- Oxytocin
- Potentiation of vasopressin action
- Nonsteroidal anti-inflammatory agents
- Carbamazepine
- Chlorpropamide
- Cyclophosphamide

- Ifosfamide
- Cisplatin
- Carboplatin
- Vincristine
- Vinblastine

Causes of SIADH Other Than Drugs

- Neoplastic disease
- Chest disorders
    - Carcinoma (bronchus, duodenum, pancreas, bladder, ureter, prostate)
    - Thymoma
    - Mesothelioma
    - Lymphoma, leukemia
    - Carcinoid
    - Bronchial adenoma
    - Pneumonia
    - Tuberculosis
    - Empyema
    - Cystic fibrosis
    - Pneumothorax
- Neurological disorders
    - Head injury, neurosurgery
    - Brain abscess or tumor
    - Meningitis, encephalitis
    - Guillain-Barré syndrome
    - Cerebral hemorrhage
    - Cavernous sinus thrombosis
    - Hydrocephalus
    - Cerebellar and cerebral atrophy
    - Shy-Drager syndrome
    - Peripheral neuropathy
    - Seizures
    - Subdural hematoma
    - Alcohol withdrawal
- Miscellaneous
    - Idiopathic
    - Psychosis
    - Porphyria
    - Abdominal surgery
- Drug-induced
    - Dopamine antagonists: phenothiazines, butyrophenones, etc.
    - Antidepressants: tricyclics, monoamineoxidase inhibitors, selective serotonin reuptake inhibitors, venlafaxine
    - Opiates
    - Antiepileptics: carbamazepine, oxcarbazipine, sodium valproate
    - 3,4-Methylenedioxymethamphetamine (MDMA; ecstasy)
    - Clofibrate
    - Cyclophosphamide
    - Chlorpropamide

Table 3-5. Diagnostic Schema for Hyponatremia.

Table 3-5. Characteristics of Different Forms of Hyponatremia Characteristics of Different Forms of Hypotonic Hyponatremia (measured serum/plasma Osmolality <280 mOsm/kG)

	Hypovolemia		Euvolemia	Hypervolemia	
Extracellular Na+	↓↓	↓↓	→	↑	↑
Total Body H20	↓	↓		↓↓	↓↓
Urinary Na+ (mmol/L)	>30 Renal loss	<30 Extra renal loss	>30	<30	>30
Common causes	• Diuretics • Addison's • Mineralocorticoid deficiency • Salt-losing nephritis • Cerebral salt wasting • Osmotic diuretics (glucose, urea, mannitol)	• Vomiting • Diarrhea • Burns • "Third Space" (e.g.pancreatitis)	• SIADH • Hypothyroidism • Glucocorticoid deficiency • Drugs	• Cardiac failure • Cirrhosis • Nephrotic syndrome	• Renal failure, or diuretic use in CHF, ascites, or nephrotic syndrome

ICD-10 CODE: Hyponatremia E87.1

ICD-10 CODE: SIADH E22.2

References:
1. Verbalis J. In Therapy of Hypoosmolar Disorders in Diseases of the kidney & urinary tract. 2007 Eighth edition Robert W. Schrier ED
2. Differential diagnosis of hyponatraemia, Chris Thompson MD FRCPIa, Tomas Berl MDb,A, Alberto Tejedor MD PhDc,B, Gudmundur Johannsson MD PhDd,CBest Practice & Research Clinical Endocrinology & Metabolism 26 Suppl. 1 (2012) S7–S15.

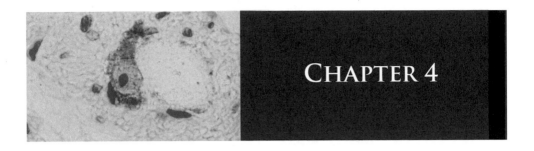

CHAPTER 4

ASSAYS, INCLUDING CPT CODES

NEUROENDOCRINE TUMORS

A COMPREHENSIVE GUIDE TO DIAGNOSIS AND MANAGEMENT

INTRODUCTION

PATIENT PREPARATION AND SPECIMEN HANDLING

For all tests it is **critical to follow exactly** the specific patient preparation and specimen handling requirements stated for each procedure listed in this catalogue. Factors such as fasting, time of collection, type of specimen, medications used, and method of shipping are vital for obtaining clinically significant information for the appropriate evaluation of a patient. Unless otherwise specified, morning, fasting specimens are preferred. In general, hormones are more sensitive to food versus neuromodulators which are insensitive to food, such as VIP, Substance P and somatostatin.

Tests that require special preservatives **must** use these special tubes for the collection of specimens to ensure that there is no loss or degradation of the hormone or peptide measured to enable accurate and meaningful determinations of the requested endocrine analytes. **Z-tube™ Preservatives, G.I. Preservative tubes, and TRH tubes are available from Inter Science Institute (ISI)** <u>**800-255-2873 or via email at: requests@interscienceinstitute.com.**</u>

A sample requisition slip is included after the index at the end of this book. Additional requisition slips are available from ISI upon request or directly from the website at interscienceinstitute.com. A requisition slip must accompany each specimen per CLIA guidelines complete with the ordering physician's address, phone and fax numbers.

Note that there are multiple methodologies, such as RIA, EIA/ELISA and GC/MS available from ISI to measure peptides and hormones. In general, whenever possible, ISI uses the most sensitive/specific method available. The assays described on the following pages are routinely performed by ISI and have been analytically and wherever possible clinically validated.

The availability of less commonly performed assays are listed at the end of the chapter and may be available on a research basis after consultation with ISI (800) 255-2873.

COLLECTION OF SPECIMENS

The majority of hormones are governed by production and clearance rates in blood and urine, which are in dynamic balance in both healthy and disease states. Since the specific hormone may not be secreted or excreted at a steady rate, urine tests are requested; thereby, eliminating or minimizing the effects of episodic secretion, determining the output of a specific analyte over a full 24-hour period, and obtaining a noninvasive specimen for analysis. The 24-hour urine sampling represents an integrated determination of the individual analytes in question taking into account the production and clearance rates. A random urine specimen is acceptable and can have a creatinine test performed to normalize the result; however, a 24-hour collection is more readily interpreted within the parameters of the reference interval. ISI has recently developed the plasma 5-HIAA test, which obviates the need for a 24-hour urine collection. (See page 131 for collection instructions.)

General Guidelines for Z-tube™, G.I. Preservative and TRH Plasma Specimens

1. ISI's preservative tubes can be used for more than one assay. The 10mL tube typically yields 3-5mL plasma. Pour off 1mL aliquots of the plasma into a non-glass shipping tube labeling each vial with the appropriate name of the test being performed by ISI.
2. Provocative stimulation or suppression tests must have time of collection noted on each vial.
3. Specimens for endocrine procedures should be obtained from patients who have been fasting overnight, preferably for 10 to 12 hours.
4. Fasting specimens should be obtained between 6:00 AM and 8:00 AM, unless otherwise stated for a particular procedure.
5. All preservative tubes are available from ISI (requests@interscienceinstitute. com or via telephone: (310) 677-3322).
6. Specimens should be collected in ISI's chilled (4° C) preservative tubes filling the 10mL tube completely. Immediately centrifuge and separate into non-glass shipping vials. Freeze plasma immediately and maintain frozen until shipped.
7. If using this plasma for more than one assay, pour off 1-2mL aliquots of the plasma labeling each vial "Z-tube plasma" and the name of the test being performed by ISI.
8. Ship frozen specimens frozen via overnight courier service. For most assays, specimens may be kept frozen for batched shipping.

Z-tube™ label:

Z™ Z-Tube Preservative
Inter Science Institute (ISI)

Special collection vacutainer tube for **Z**-Tube specimens. Instructions: DRAW SPECIMEN INTO COOLED 4° C TUBE FILLING TUBE COMPLETELY, IF POSSIBLE; CENTRIFUGE IMMEDIATELY, TRANSFER PLASMA TO PLASTIC VIAL AND FREEZE IMMEDIATELY. SHIP FROZEN ON DRY ICE.
ISI's **Z**-tube to be used specifically for ISI's Neuroendocrine peptides: Pancreastatin; Neurokinin A; Substance P; Neurotensin; Neuropeptide Y; Pancreatic Polypeptide (PP); 5-HIAA (plasma).

Z™-Collection Plasma Tube

Use the Z-tube™ for these assays:

- 5-HIAA (Plasma)
- Neurokinin A (Substance K)
- Neuropeptide Y (NPY)
- Neurotensin
- Pancreastatin
- Substance P

G.I. Preservative tube label:

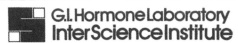

G.I. Hormone Laboratory
InterScienceInstitute

SPECIAL COLLECTION VACUTAINER TUBE FOR GI SPECIMENS
INSTRUCTIONS: DRAW SPECIMEN INTO COOLED
4°C TUBE: CENTRIFUGE **IMMEDIATELY** TRANSFER PLASMA TO
PLASTIC VIAL AND FREEZE **IMMEDIATELY**. SHIP FROZEN. store at 4°C

Use the G.I. Preservative tube for these assays:

- Adiponectin
- Amylin
- Bombesin
- Cholecystokinin (CCK)
- Gastric Inhibitory Polypeptide (GIP)
- Gastrin Releasing Peptide (GRP)
- Ghrelin, Total
- Glucagon
- GLP-1, Total
- Leptin, Total
- Neuropeptide K
- Secretin
- Somatostatin
- Vasoactive Intestinal Polypeptide (VIP)

TRH Preservative tube label:

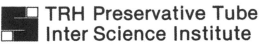

TRH Preservative Tube
Inter Science Institute

SPECIAL COLLECTION VACUTAINER TUBE. INSTRUCTIONS: DRAW
SPECIMEN INTO COOLED 4°C TUBE. CENTRIFUGE **IMMEDIATELY**.
TRANSFER PLASMA TO PLASTIC VIAL AND FREEZE **IMMEDIATELY**.
SHIP FROZEN. (Avoid hemolysis as TRH is inactivated.) store at 4°C.

The TRH Preservative tube is only used for the Thyrotropin Releasing Hormone (TRH) assay performed by ISI.

General Guidelines for other EDTA Plasma or Serum Specimens

1. Specimens for endocrine procedures preferably should be obtained from patients who have been fasting overnight for 10 to 12 hours.
2. Fasting specimens should be obtained between 6:00 AM and 8:00 AM, unless otherwise stated for a particular procedure; if this not possible, six to eight hours postprandial is adequate.
3. The patient should discontinue medications that may affect hormone levels for at least 48 hours prior to collection under the guidance and consent of his or her physician (See special instructions for Octreotide [Sandostatin®] in Chapter 4 on page [to be added once document is paginated]).
4. Some tests require the use of the preservative collection tubes as noted above to obtain valid analysis of specimens. Preservative tubes are available from ISI via email at requests@interscienceinstitute.com or via telephone: (800) ALL-CURE or (310) 677-3322. (See specific pages for preservative tube collection requirements.)
5. For measurement of Octreotide (Sandostatin®) or Lanreotide (Somatuline Depot®) levels, specimen should be collected the day before the next LAR injection is administered.
6. Ship specimens frozen via overnight courier service unless otherwise noted under each specific test.

Standard EDTA preservative tubes or serum or serum separator tubes (SSTs) can be used for these assays:

- C-Peptide
- Calcitonin
- Chromogranin A (CgA)
- Gastrin
- Growth Hormone (GH)
- Growth Hormone – Releasing Hormone (GH-RH)
- Lanreotide
- Melanocyte Stimulating Hormone-Alpha, Beta or Gamma (MSH)
- Melatonin
- Motilin
- Octreotide
- Pancreatic Polypeptide (PP)
- Pepsinogen I
- Pepsinogen II
- Prostaglandins (PG D2, PG E1, PG E2, PG F2-Alpha)

General Guidelines for Collection of a 24-Hour Urine Specimen

1. Begin urine collection after discarding first morning voiding.
2. Collect all other urine voidings during the next 24 hours, including the first AM voiding the next day.
3. Record the 24-hour volume.
4. Mix urine well and remove appropriate aliquot to submit for analysis.
5. Boric acid tablets may be added to urine to reduce bacterial growth.
6. Ensure that urine procedures stating **"Do not acidify urine"** are <u>not</u> collected with hydrochloric or acetic acid.
7. If possible, urine should be refrigerated during collection and shipped frozen to avoid leakage. Provide total volume per 24 hours.
8. If a 24-hour volume is not available, a random urine specimen is acceptable and can have a creatinine test performed to normalize the result; however, a 24-hour collection is more readily interpreted within the parameters of the reference interval that is listed per 24 hours.

General Guidelines for Collection of a Fecal Sample

Collect 100 mg (size of dime) of formed stool and store at −20°C. Stool specimens are stable for 7 days when refrigerated. Note on request slip if sample has watery diarrhea consistency, as concentration levels may be decreased due to the dilution factor. See individual test (Elastase, Pancreatic - fecal) for specific requirements.

Special Fluids

For special fluids, such as CSF, vitreous fluid, peritoneal fluid, synovial fluid, contact ISI for requirements and special handling instructions.
Submit 2-3mL, if possible, for each assay requested and ship frozen in dry ice.
Minimum specimen size is 1mL.

Shipping Instructions

To maintain specimen integrity, ship specimens frozen in dry ice via overnight courier, such as Federal Express®. Some specimens are stable ambient (room temperature) for up to three days. See individual tests for stability information and required shipping temperatures.

Federal Express shipping address:

Inter Science Institute
944 W. Hyde Park Blvd.
Inglewood CA 90302
(310) 677-3322

Contact Information for Inter Science Institute

Toll free: (800) 255-2873 (USA only)
Local: (310) 677-3322 (outside the USA)
Email: requests@interscienceinstitute.com

ADIPONECTIN*

Reference Interval

Reference range is listed on individual patient reports.

Procedure

Adiponectin is measured by direct radioimmunoassay.

Patient Preparation

The patient should fast for 10 to 12 hours, if possible, prior to collection of specimen. Insulin, medications, or other factors that affect insulin or amylin secretion should be discontinued, if possible, for at least 48 hours prior to collection of specimen.

Specimen Collection

Collect 10mL blood directly into ISI's G.I. Preservative tube and separate as soon as possible. Freeze plasma immediately after separation. Special G.I. Preservative tubes are available from ISI. Minimum specimen size is 1mL.

Important Precaution

Adiponectin specimens must be collected using ISI's G.I. Preservative tube. No other methods of collection are acceptable.

Special Specimens

For special fluids, such as CSF, vitreous fluid, peritoneal fluid, synovial fluid, contact ISI for requirements and special handling instructions.

Shipping Instructions

Ship specimens frozen in dry ice.

References
1. Lieb DC, Parson HK, Mamikunian G, Vinik AI. Cardiac autonomic imbalance in newly diagnosed and established diabetes is associated with markers of adipose tissue inflammation. Exp Diabetes Res. Research Article. 2012;2012:878760.Epub.2011 Nov 1.
2. Fu Y, Luo N, Klein RL, et al. Adiponectin promotes adipocyte differentiation, insulin sensitivity, and lipid accumulation: potential role in autoregulation of adipocyte metabolism and adipose mass. J Lipid Res. 2005. July;46(7):1369-79.
3. Brame LA, Considine RV, Yamauchi M, et al. Insulin and endothelin in the acute regulation of adiponectin in vivo in humans. Obes Res. Mar 2005;13(3):582-8.
4. Milewicz A, Zatonska K, Demissie M, et al. Serum adiponectin concentration and cardiovascular risk factors in climacteric women. Gynecol Endocrinol. 2005;Feb;20(2):68-73.
5. Ballantyne CM, Nambi V. Markers of inflammation and their clinical significance. Atheroscler Suppl. 2005; 2 May;6(2):21-9.
6. Matsuzawa Y. Adiponectin: identification, physiology and clinical relevance in metabolic and vascular disease. Atheroscler Suppl. 2005;May;6(2):7-14.

* In preparation

CPT Code:
Unspecified Quantitative Immunoassay 83519

AMYLIN

Reference Interval

Reference range is listed on individual patient reports.

Procedure

Amylin is measured by direct radioimmunoassay.

Patient Preparation

The patient should fast for 10 to 12 hours, if possible, prior to collection of specimen. Insulin, medications, or other factors that affect insulin or amylin secretion should be discontinued, if possible, for at least 48 hours prior to collection of specimen.

Specimen Collection

Collect 10mL blood directly into ISI's G.I. Preservative tube and separate as soon as possible. Freeze plasma immediately after separation. Special G.I. Preservative tubes are available from ISI. Minimum specimen size is 1mL.

Important Precaution

Amylin specimens must be collected using ISI's G.I. Preservative tube. No other methods of collection are acceptable.

Special Specimens

For special fluids, such as CSF, vitreous fluid, peritoneal fluid, synovial fluid, contact ISI for requirements and special handling instructions.

Shipping Instructions

Ship specimens frozen in dry ice.

References
1. Sanke T, Hanabusa T, Nakano Y, et al. Plasma islet amyloid polypeptide (amylin) levels and their responses to oral glucose in type 2 (non-insulin-dependent) diabetic patients. Diabetologia.1991;34:129-32.
2. Hartter E, Svoboda T, Lydvik B, et al. Basal and stimulated plasma levels of pancreatic amylin indicate its co-secretion with insulin in humans. Diabetologia.1991;34:52-4.
3. Bronsky J, Prusa R. Amylin fasting plasma levels are decreased in patients with osteoporosis. Osteoporos Int.2004;15(3):243-
4. Samonina GE, Kopylova GN, Lukjanzeva GV, et al. Antiulcer effects of amylin: a review. Pathophysiology.2004;11(1):1-6.
5. Ludvik B, Thomaseth K, Nolan JJ, et al. Inverse relation between amylin and glucagon secretion in healthy and diabetic human subjects. Eur J Clin Invest. 2003;33(4):316-22.

CPT Code:
Unspecified Quantitative Immunoassay 83519

BOMBESIN

Reference Interval

50–250 pg/mL

Procedure

Bombesin is measured by direct radioimmunoassay.

Patient Preparation

The patient should fast for 10 to 12 hours prior to collection of specimen. Antacid medications and medications that affect intestinal motility should be discontinued, if possible, for at least 48 hours prior to collection of specimen.

Specimen Collection

Collect 10mL blood directly into ISI's G.I. Preservative tube and separate as soon as possible. Freeze plasma immediately after separation. Special G.I. Preservative tubes are available from ISI. Minimum specimen size is 1mL.

Important Precaution

Bombesin specimens must be collected using ISI's G.I. Preservative tube. No other methods of collection are acceptable.

Special Specimens

For special fluids, such as CSF, vitreous fluid, peritoneal fluid, synovial fluid, contact ISI for requirements and special handling instructions.

Shipping Instructions

Ship specimens frozen in dry ice.

References
1. Mahmoud S, Palaszynski E, Fiskum G, et al. Small cell lung cancer bombesin receptors are antagonized by reduced peptide analogs. Life Sci. 1989;44(5):367-73.
2. Tache Y, Gunion M. Central nervous system action of bombesin to inhibit gastrin acid secretion. Life Sci.1985;15 Jul;37(2):115-23.
3. Yegen BC. Bombesin-like peptides: candidates as diagnostic and therapeutic tools. Curr Pharm. 2003;Dec;9(12):1013-22.
4. Zhou J, Chen J, Mokotoff M, et al. Bombesin/gastrin-releasing peptide receptor: a potential target for antibody-mediated therapy of small cell lung cancer. Clin Cancer Res. 2003;9(13):4953-60.
5. Mandragos C, Moukas M, Amygdalou A, et al. Gastrointestinal hormones and short-term nutritional schedules in critically ill patients. Hepatogastroenterology.2003;50(53):1442-5.
6. Scott N, Millward E, Cartwright EJ, et al. Gastrin releasing peptide and gastrin releasing peptide receptor expression in gastrointestinal carcinoid tumours. J Clin Pathol. 2004; 57(2):189-92.

CPT Code:
Unspecified Quantitative Immunoassay 83519

C-PEPTIDE

Reference Interval

0.9–4.2 ng/mL

Procedure

C-peptide is measured by direct radioimmunoassay.

Patient Preparation

The patient should not be on any insulin therapy nor take medications that influence insulin levels, if possible, for at least 48 hours prior to collection of specimen.

Specimen Collection

Collect 3mL of serum or EDTA plasma and separate as soon as possible. Freeze serum or plasma immediately after separation. Minimum specimen size is 1mL.

Special Specimens

For special fluids, such as CSF, vitreous fluid, peritoneal fluid, synovial fluid, contact ISI for requirements and special handling instructions.

Shipping Instructions

Ship specimens frozen in dry ice.

References
1. Myrick JE, Gunter EW, Maggio VL, et al. An improved radioimmunoassay of C-peptide and its application in a multiyear study. Clin Chem. 1989;35:7-12.
2. Ludvigsson J. Methodological aspects of C-peptide measurements. Acta Med Scand (Suppl). 671:53-9, 1983.
3. Bell DS, Ovalle F. The role of C-peptide levels in screening for latent autoimmune diabetes in adults. Am J Ther. 2004;11(4):308-11.
4. Jazet IM, Pijl H, Frolich M, et al. Factors predicting the blood glucose lowering effect of a 30-day very low calorie diet in obese type 2 diabetic patients. Diabet Med. 22(1):52-5, 2005.
5. Ovalle F, Bell DS. Effect of rosiglitazone versus insulin on the pancreatic beta-cell function of subjects with type 2 diabetes. Diabetes Care. 2005; 27(11):2585-9.
6. Landin-Olsson M. Latent autoimmune diabetes in adults. Ann NY Acad Sci. 2002;Apr;958:112-6.
7. Torn C. C-peptide and autoimmune markers in diabetes. Clin Lab. 2003;49(1-2):1-10.

CPT Code:
C-Peptide, insulin induced 80432
C-Peptide 84681

CHOLECYSTOKININ (CCK)

Reference Interval

Up to 80 pg/mL

Procedure

CCK is measured by direct radioimmunoassay.

Patient Preparation

The patient should fast for 10 to 12 hours prior to collection of specimen. Antacid medications and medications that affect intestinal motility should be discontinued, if possible, for at least 48 hours prior to collection of specimen.

Specimen Collection

Collect 10mL blood directly into ISI's G.I. Preservative tube and separate as soon as possible. Freeze plasma immediately after separation. Special G.I. Preservative tubes are available from ISI. Minimum specimen size is 1mL.

Important Precaution

CCK specimens must be collected using ISI's G.I. Preservative tube. No other methods of collection are acceptable.

Special Specimens

For special fluids, such as CSF, vitreous fluid, peritoneal fluid, synovial fluid, contact ISI for requirements and special handling instructions.

Shipping Instructions

Ship specimens frozen in dry ice.

References
1. Nakano I, Funakoshi A, Shinozaki H, et al. Plasma cholecystokinin and pancreatic polypeptide responses after ingestion of a liquid test meal rich in medium-chain fatty acids in patients with chronic pancreatitis. Am J Clin Nutr. 1989;Feb;49(2):247-51.
2. Chang T, Chey WY. Radioimmunoassay of cholecystokinin. Dig Dis Sci. May;28(5):456-68, 1983.
3. Rehfeld JF. Clinical endocrinology and metabolism. Cholecystokinin. Best Pract Res Clin Endocrinol Metab. 2004;18(4):569-86.

CPT Code:
Unspecified Quantitative Immunoassay 83519

CHROMOGRANIN A (CgA)

Reference Interval

Up to 40 ng/mL

Procedure

CgA is measured by direct radioimmunoassay/enzyme immunoassay (EIA)/ELISA.

Patient Preparation

The patient should fast for 10 to 12 hours prior to collection of specimen. Antacid medications and medications that affect intestinal motility should be discontinued, if possible, for at least 48 hours prior to collection of specimen.

Specimen Collection

Collect 10mL blood in an EDTA or red-topped tube. 3mL plasma or serum should be separated as soon as possible. Specimen can be shipped refrigerated, or frozen in dry ice.

Important Precaution

Draw sample first thing in the morning because of the diurnal variation. When serial measurements are made, draw samples at the same time each day.

Special Specimens

For special fluids, such as CSF, vitreous fluid, peritoneal fluid, synovial fluid, contact ISI for requirements and special handling instructions.

Shipping Instructions

Ship specimens frozen in dry ice.

References
1. Woltering EA, Hilton RS, Zolfoghary CM, et al Validation of serum versus plasma measurements of chromogranin A levels in patients with carcinoid tumors: lack of correlation between absolute chromogranin A levels and symptom frequency. Pancreas2006;33(3):250-4.
2. Vinik AI, Silva MP, Woltering EA, et al. Biochemical testing for neuroendocrine tumors (NETs). Pancreas. 38(8): 876-879, 2009. Review Erratum In: 2010;39(1):117.
3. Öberg K, Kvols L, Caplin M, et al. Consensus report on the use of somatostatin analogs for the management of neuroendocrine tumors of the gastroenteropancreatic system. Ann Oncol. 2004; 15:966-73.
   • Nehar D, Olivieri S, Claustrat B, et al. Interest of Chromogranin A for diagnosis and follow-up of endocrine tumours. Clin Endocrinol (Oxf). 2004; 60(5):644-52.
   • Viola KV, Sosa JA. Current advances in the diagnosis and treatment of pancreatic endocrine tumors. Curr Opin Oncol. 2005;17(1):24-7.
4. d'Herbomez M, Gouze V, Huglo D, et al. Chromogranin A assay and 131I-MIBG scintigraphy for diagnosis and follow-up of pheochromocytoma. J Nucl Med. 2001;Jul;42(7):993-7.
5. Giusti M, Sidoti M, Augeri C, et al. Effect of short-term treatment with low dosages of the proton-pump inhibitor omeprazole on serum chromogranin A levels in man. Eur J Endocrinol. 2004;Mar;150(3):299-303.
6. Biausque F, Jaboureck O, Devos P, et al. Clinical significant of serum chromogranin A levels for diagnosing pheochromocytoma in hypertensive patients. Arch Mal Coeur Vaiss. 2003;Jul-Aug;96(7-8):780-3.
7. Giampaolo B, Angelica M, Antonio S. Chromogranin 'A' in normal subjects, essential hypertensives and adrenalectomized patients. Clin Endocrinol. 2002;Jul;57(1):41-50.

CPT Code:
CgA 86316

ELASTASE, PANCREATIC (SERUM)

Reference Interval

Up to 3.5 ng/mL

Procedure

Elastase is measured by direct radioimmunoassay.

Patient Preparation

The patient should fast for 10 to 12 hours prior to collection of specimen. Medications that affect pancreatic activity should be discontinued, if possible, for at least 48 hours prior to collection of specimen.

Specimen Collection

Collect 3mL serum and separate as soon as possible. Freeze serum immediately after separation. Minimum specimen size is 1mL.

Special Specimens

For special fluids, such as CSF, vitreous, peritoneal fluid, synovial fluid, contact ISI for requirements and special handling instructions. (See alternate matrix: Elastase-1, Fecal.)

Shipping Instructions

Ship specimens frozen in dry ice.

References
1. Wortsman J, Matsuoka LY, Kueppers F. Elastase inhibitory activity in serum of patients with thyroid dysfunction. Clin Chem. 1991; 37:108-10.
2. Geokas MC, Brodrick JW, Johnson JH, et al. Pancreatic elastase in human serum. Determination by radioimmunoassay. J Biol Chem. 1977;10 Jan; 252(1):61-7.

CPT Code:
Pancreatic Elastase I 82656

ELASTASE-1 (EL1), FECAL

Reference Interval

Normal: 200 to >500 µg/g stool
Moderate to mild pancreatic insufficiency: 100–200 µg/g stool
Severe exocrine pancreatic insufficiency: <100 µg/g stool

Procedure

EL1 is measured by a monoclonal antibody specific only to human pancreatic EL1 employing ELISA.

Patient Preparation

No special patient preparation is required, because substitution therapy has no influence on the specific fecal EL1 levels.

Specimen Collection

Collect 100 mg formed stool and store at –20°C. Stool specimens are stable for 7 days when refrigerated. Minimum specimen size is 20 mg of formed stool. Note if sample has watery diarrhea consistency the concentration of EL1 may be decreased due to the dilution factor.

Special Specimens

Stool is the only appropriate specimen for this test. (See alternate matrix: Elastase, Pancreatic - Serum).

Shipping Instructions

Ship specimens frozen in dry ice.

References
1. Hahn JU, Bochnig S, Kerner W, et al. A new fecal elastase 1 test using polyclonal antibodies for the detection of exocrine pancreatic insufficiency. Pancreas. 2005;Mar;30(2):189-91.
2. Luth S, Teyssen S, Forssmann K, et al. Fecal elastase-1 determination:'gold standard' of indirect pancreatic function tests? Scand J Gastroenterol. 2001;Oct;36(10):1092-9.
3. Gullo L, Ventrucci M, Tomassetti P, et al. Fecal elastase 1 determination in chronic pancreatitis. Dig Dis Sci. 1999;Jan;44(1):210-3.

CPT Code:
Fecal Elastase 82656

GASTRIC INHIBITORY POLYPEPTIDE (GIP; GLUCOSE-DEPENDENT INSULINOTROPIC PEPTIDE)

Reference Interval

Fasting:	Up to 50 pg/mL
Post-Prandial:	110 - 720 pg/mL

Procedure

GIP is measured by direct radioimmunoassay.

Patient Preparation

The patient should fast for 10 to 12 hours prior to collection of specimen. Antacid medications and medications that affect intestinal motility or insulin secretion should be discontinued, if possible, for at least 48 hours prior to collection of specimen.

Specimen Collection

Collect 10mL blood directly into ISI's G.I. Preservative tube and separate as soon as possible. Freeze plasma immediately after separation. Special G.I. Preservative tubes are available from ISI. Minimum specimen size is 1mL.

Important Precaution

GIP specimens must be collected using ISI's G.I. Preservative tube. No other methods of collection are acceptable.

Special Specimens

For special fluids, such as CSF, vitreous fluid, peritoneal fluid, synovial fluid, contact ISI for requirements and special handling instructions.

Shipping Instructions

Ship specimens frozen in dry ice.

References
1. Krarup T. Immunoreactive gastric inhibitory polypeptide. Endocr Rev.1988;Feb;9(1):122-34.
2. Sarson DL, Bryant MG, Bloom SR. A radioimmunoassay of gastric inhibitory polypeptide in human plasma. J Endocrinol. 1980;Jun;85(3):487-96.
3. Thomas RP, Hellmich MR, Townsend CM Jr, et al. Role of gastrointestinal hormones in the proliferation of normal and neoplastic tissues. Endocr Rev. 2003;24(5):571-99.
4. Calhoun K, Toth-Fejel S, Cheek J, et al. Serum peptide profiles in patients with carcinoid tumors. Am J Surg. 2003; 186(1):28-3.
5. Meier JJ, Nauck, MA. Clinical endocrinology and metabolism. Glucose-dependent insulinotropic polypeptide/gastric inhibitory polypeptide. Best Pract Res Clin Endocrinol Metab. 2004;18(4):587-606.
6. Nauck MA, Baller B, Meier JJ. Gastric inhibitory polypeptide and glucagon-like peptide-1 in the pathogenesis of type 2 diabetes. Diabetes. 2004;53(Suppl 3):S190-6.

CPT Code:
Unspecified Quantitative Immunoassay 83519

GASTRIN

Reference Interval

Up to 75 pg/mL

Procedure

Gastrin is measured by direct radioimmunoassay.

Patient Preparation

The patient should fast for 10 to 12 hours prior to collection of specimen. Proton pump inhibitors (PPIs) and antacid medications should be discontinued, if possible, for at least 48 hours prior to collection of specimen.

Specimen Collection

Collect 3mL serum or EDTA plasma and separate as soon as possible. Freeze serum or plasma immediately after separation. Minimum specimen size is 1mL.

Special Specimens

For special fluids, such as CSF, vitreous fluid, peritoneal fluid, synovial fluid, contact ISI for requirements and special handling instructions.

Shipping Instructions

Ship specimens frozen in dry ice.

References
1. Raines D, Chester M, Diebold AE, et al. A prospective evaluation of the effect of chronic proton pump inhibitor use on plasma biomarker levels in humans. Pancreas. 2012;41(4):508-511.
2. Tetsuhide I, Hisato I, and Jensen R. Serum Pancreastatin: the long sought universal, sensitive, specific tumor marker for neuroendocrine tumors? Editorial. Pancreas. 2012;41(4):505-507.
3. Bostwick DG, Bensch KG. Gastrin releasing peptide in human neuroendocrine tumors. J Pathol. 1985;Dec;147(4):237-44.
4. Walsh JH, Isenberg JI, Ansfield J, et al. Clearance and acid-stimulating action of human big and little gastrins in duodenal ulcer subjects. J Clin Invest. 1976;May;57(5):1125-31.
5. Dockray G, Dimaline R, Varro A. Gastrin: old hormone, new functions. Pflugers Arch. 2005;449(4): 344-55.
6. Mignon, M. Diagnostic and therapeutic strategies in Zollinger-Ellison syndrome associated with multiple endocrine neoplasia type I (MEN-I): experience of the Zollinger-Ellison Syndrome Research Group: Bichat 1958-1999. Bull Acad Nat Med. 2003;187(7):1249-58.

CPT Code:
Gastrin 82938–82941 after secretion stimulation

GASTRIN-RELEASING PEPTIDE (GRP)

Reference Interval

10–80 pg/mL

Procedure

GRP is measured by direct radioimmunoassay.

Patient Preparation

The patient should fast for 10 to 12 hours prior to collection of specimen. Proton pump inhibitors (PPIs) and antacid medications and medications that affect intestinal motility should be discontinued, if possible, for at least 48 hours prior to collection of specimen.

Specimen Collection

Collect 10mL blood directly into ISI's G.I. Preservative tube and separate as soon as possible. Freeze plasma immediately after separation. Special G.I. Preservative tubes are available from ISI. Minimum specimen size is 1mL.

Important Precaution

GRP specimens must be collected using ISI's G.I. Preservative tube. No other methods of collection are acceptable.

Special Specimens

For special fluids, such as CSF, vitreous fluid, peritoneal fluid, synovial fluid, contact ISI for requirements and special handling instructions.

Shipping Instructions

Ship specimens frozen in dry ice.

References

1. Bostwick DG, Bensch KG. Gastrin releasing peptide in human neuroendocrine tumors. J Pathol. 1985;Dec;147(4):237-44.
2. Carney DN, Cuttitta F, Moody TW, et al. Selective stimulation of small cell lung cancer clonal growth by bombesin and gastrin releasing peptide. Cancer Res. 19871;Feb;47(3):821-5.
3. Thomas RP, Hellmich MR, Townsend CM Jr, et al. Role of gastrointestinal hormones in the proliferation of normal and neoplastic tissues. Endocr Rev. 2003;24(5):571-99.
4. Calhoun K, Toth-Fejel S, Cheek J, et al. Serum peptide profiles in patients with carcinoid tumors. Am J Surg. 2003;186(1):28-31.
5. Sunday ME. Pulmonary neuroendocrine cells and lung development. Endocr Pathol. 1996;7(3):173-201.

CPT Code:
Unspecified Quantitative Immunoassay 83519

GHRELIN, TOTAL

Reference Interval

520 – 700 pg/mL

Procedure

Ghrelin is measured by direct radioimmunoassay.

Patient Preparation

Patient should be fasting for 10 - 12 hours prior to collection of specimens. Patient should not be on any medications or supplements that may influence cholecystokinin (CCK), growth hormone, insulin and/or somatostatin levels, if possible, for at least 48 hours prior to collection.

Specimen Collection

Collect 10mL blood directly into ISI's G.I. Preservative tube and separate as soon as possible. Freeze plasma immediately after separation. Special G.I. Preservative tubes are available from ISI. Minimum specimen size is 1mL.

Important Precaution

Ghrelin specimens must be collected using ISI's G.I. Preservative tube. No other methods of collection are acceptable.

Special Specimens

For special fluids, such as CSF, vitreous fluid, peritoneal fluid, synovial fluid, contact ISI for requirements and special handling instructions.

Shipping Instructions

Ship specimens frozen in dry ice.

References
1. Butler MG, Bittel DC and Talebizadeh Z. Plasma peptide YY and ghrelin levels in infants and children with prader-willi syndrome. J Ped Endocrinol Metab. 2004;Sep; 17(9): 1177-1184.
2. Shiiya T, Nakazato, Mizuta M et al. Plasma ghrelin levels in lean and obese humans and the effect of glucose on ghrelin secretion. J Clin Endocrinol Metab. 2002;Jan; 87(1): 240-244.

CPT Code:
Unspecified Quantitative Immunoassay 83519

GLUCAGON

Reference Intervals

Age (year)	Range (pg/mL)
20–29	20–180
30–39	10–250
40–49	40–215
50–59	75–170
60–69	50–270

Procedure

Glucagon is measured by direct radioimmunoassay.

Patient Preparation

The patient should fast for 10 to 12 hours prior to collection of specimen. The patient should not take any medications that influence insulin secretion or intestinal motility, if possible, for at least 48 hours prior to collection of specimen.

Specimen Collection

Collect 10mL blood directly into ISI's G.I. Preservative tube and separate as soon as possible. Freeze plasma immediately after separation. Special G.I. Preservative tubes are available from ISI. Minimum specimen size is 1mL.

Important Precaution

Glucagon specimens must be collected using ISI's G.I. Preservative tube. No other methods of collection are acceptable.

Special Specimens

For special fluids, such as CSF, vitreous fluid, peritoneal fluid, synovial fluid, contact ISI for requirements and special handling instructions.

Shipping Instructions

Ship specimens frozen in dry ice.

References
1. Philippe J, Mojsov S, Drucker DJ, et al. Proglucagon processing in a rat islet cell line resembles phenotype of intestine rather than pancreas. Endocrinology. 1986;Dec;119(6):2833-9.
2. Weir GC, Mojsov S, Hendrick GK, et al. Glucagonlike peptide I (7-37) actions on endocrine pancreas. Diabetes. 1989;Mar;38(3):338-42.
3. van Beek AP, de Haas ER, van Vloten WA, et al. The glucagonoma syndrome and necrolytic migratory erythema: a clinical review. Eur J Endocrinol. 2004; 151(5):531-7.

CPT Codes:
Glucagon 82943 • Tolerance Panel; for pheochromocytoma 80424 (Must include Catecholamines, fractionated 82394 x2 • Tolerance Panel; for insulinoma 80422 (Must include Glucose 82947 x3, Insulin 83525 x3

GLUCAGON-LIKE PEPTIDE 1 (GLP-1), TOTAL

Reference Interval

Fasting:	Non-Detectable to less than 50 pmol/L
Post-Prandial:	2 to 5 times greater concentration than fasting specimens.

Procedure

GLP-1, Total is measured by direct radioimmunoassay.

Patient Preparation

The patient should fast for 10 to 12 hours prior to collection of specimen. Antacid medications and medications that affect intestinal motility or insulin secretion should be discontinued, if possible, for at least 48 hours prior to collection of specimen.

Specimen Collection

Collect 10mL blood directly into ISI's G.I. Preservative tube and separate as soon as possible. Freeze plasma immediately after separation. Special G.I. Preservative tubes are available from ISI. Minimum specimen size is 1mL.

Important Precautions

GLP-1 specimens must be collected using ISI's G.I. Preservative tube. No other methods of collection are acceptable.

Special Specimens

For special fluids, such as CSF, vitreous fluid, peritoneal fluid, synovial fluid, contact ISI for requirements and special handling instructions.

Shipping Instructions

Ship specimens frozen in dry ice.

References
1. Philippe J, Mojsov S, Drucker DJ, et al. Proglucagon processing in a rat islet cell line resembles phenotype of intestine rather than pancreas. Endocrinology. 1986;Dec;119(6):2833-9.
2. Weir GC, Mojsov S, Hendrick GK, et al. Glucagonlike peptide I (7-37) actions on endocrine pancreas. Diabetes. 1989;Mar;38(3):338-42.
3. Meier JJ, Nauck MA. Clinical endocrinology and metabolism. Glucose-dependent insulinotropic polypeptide/gastric inhibitory polypeptide. Best Pract Res Clin Endocrinol Metab. 2004;18(4):587-606.
4. Nauck MA, Baller B, Meier JJ. Gastric inhibitory polypeptide and glucagon-like peptide-1 in the pathogenesis of type 2 diabetes. Diabetes. 2004;53(Suppl 3):S190-6.
5. Drucker DJ. Glucagon-like peptides. Diabetes. 1998;47(2):159-69.
6. Drucker DJ. Biological actions and therapeutic potential of the glucagon-like peptides. Gastroenterology. 2002;122(2):531-44.
7. Lovshin J, Drucker DJ. Synthesis, secretion and biological actions of the glucagon-like peptides. Pediatr Diabetes. 2000;1(1):49-57.

CPT Code:
Unspecified Quantitative Immunoassay 83519

GROWTH HORMONE (GH, SOMATOTROPIN)

Reference Interval

Children:	Up to 20 ng/mL
Adults:	Up to 10 ng/mL

Procedure

GH is measured by direct radioimmunoassay.

Patient Preparation

The patient should not be on any insulin therapy nor take ACTH or gonadotropin medication, if possible, for at least 48 hours prior to collection of specimen.

Specimen Collection

Collect 3mL serum or EDTA plasma and separate as soon as possible. Freeze plasma immediately after separation. Minimum specimen size is 1mL.

Special Specimens

For special fluids, such as CSF, vitreous fluid, peritoneal fluid, synovial fluid, contact ISI for requirements and special handling instructions.

Shipping Instructions

Ship specimens at room temperature, refrigerated, or frozen in dry ice.

References
1. Word RA, Odom MJ, Byrd W, et al. The effect of gonadotropin-releasing hormone Agonists on growth hormone secretion in adult premenopausal women. Fertil Steril. 1990;Jul;54(1):73-8.
2. Strasburger C, Barnard G, Toldo L, et al. Somatotropin as measured by a two-site time-resolved immunofluorometric assay. Clin Chem. 1989;Jun;35(6):913-7.
3. Sheppard MC. Growth hormone—from molecule to mortality. Clin Med. 2004;4(5):437-40.

CPT Code:
Growth Hormone 83003

GROWTH HORMONE–RELEASING HORMONE (GH-RH)

Reference Interval

5–18 pg/mL

Procedure

GH-RH is measured by direct radioimmunoassay.

Patient Preparation

The patient should not take any medications that influence pituitary secretion (such as arginine), if possible, for at least 48 hours prior to collection of specimen.

Specimen Collection

Collect 3mL serum or EDTA plasma and separate as soon as possible. Freeze serum or plasma immediately after separation. Minimum specimen size is 1mL.

Special Specimens

For special fluids, such as CSF, vitreous fluid, peritoneal fluid, synovial fluid, contact ISI for requirements and special handling instructions.

Shipping Instructions

Ship specimens frozen in dry ice.

References
1. Vance ML. Growth-hormone releasing hormone. Clin Chem. 1990;36:415-20.
2. Sopwith AM, Penny ES, Grossman A, et al. Normal circulating growth hormone releasing factor (hGRF) concentrations in patients with functional hypothalamic hGRF deficiency. Clin Endocrinol (Oxf). 1986; 24:395-400.
3. Groot K, Csernus VJ, Pinski J, et al. Development of a radioimmunoassay for some agonists of growth hormone-releasing hormone. Int J Pept Protein Res. 1993;41(2):162-8.
4. DeLellis RA, Xia L. Paraneoplastic endocrine syndromes: a review. Endocr Pathol. 2003;14(4):303-17.

CPT Code:
Growth Hormone– Releasing Hormone 83519

HISTAMINE

Reference Interval

Up to 100 ng/dL

Procedure

Histamine is measured by direct radioimmunoassay.

Patient Preparation

The patient should not take any antihistamine medication, if possible, for at least 48 hours prior to collection of specimen.

Specimen Collection

Collect 3mL EDTA plasma and separate as soon as possible. Freeze plasma immediately after separation. Minimum specimen size is 1 mL. Neither serum nor whole blood are acceptable specimen types for this assay.

Special Specimens

For special fluids, such as CSF, vitreous fluid, peritoneal fluid, synovial fluid, contact ISI for requirements and special handling instructions.

Shipping Instructions

Ship specimens frozen in dry ice.

References
1. Marquardt DL. Histamine. Clin Rev Allergy. 1983; Sep;1(3):343-51.
2. Harsing LG Jr, Nagashima H, Duncalf D, et al. Determination of histamine concentrations in plasma by liquid chromatography/electrochemistry. Clin Chem (Oxf). 1986; Oct;32(10):1823-7.

CPT Code:
Histamine 83088

5-HIAA (5-HYDROXYINDOLEACETIC ACID), PLASMA*

Reference Interval

Up to 22 ng/mL

Procedure

5-HIAA plasma is measured by GC-MS/MS.

Patient Preparation

The patient should fast for 8 hours prior to collection of specimen.

Specimen Collection

Collect 10mL blood directly into ISI's Z-tube™ Preservative and separate as soon as possible. Freeze plasma immediately after separation. Special Z-tube™ Preservatives are available from ISI. Minimum specimen size is 1mL.

Important Precaution

5-HIAA plasma specimens must be collected using ISI's Z-tube™ Preservative. No other methods of collection are acceptable.

Special Specimens

*Frozen Z-tube™ plasma is the only acceptable sample type for this assay.

Shipping Instructions

Ship specimens frozen in dry ice.

References
1. Tellez MR, Mamikunian G, O'Dorisio TM et al. A single fasting plasma 5-HIAA value correlates with 24-hour urinary 5-HIAA values and other biomarkers in midgut neuroendocrine tumors (NETs). Pancreas. 2013:42(3): 405-410.
2. Cai H-L, Zhu R-H, Li H-D, et al. MultiSimplex optimization of chromatographic separation and dansyl derivatization conditions in the ultra performance liquid chromatography-tandem mass spectrometry analysis of neurotransmitters in human urine. J Chromato B 2011;879:1993-1999.
3. Gonzalez RR, Fernandez RF, Vidal JLM et al. Development and validation of an ultra-high performance liquid chromatography-tandem mass spectrometry (UHPLC-MS/MS) method for the simultaneous determination of neurotransmitters in rat brain samples. J Neuro Meth 2011;198: 187-194.
4. Stephanson N, Helander A, Beck O. Alcohol biomarker analysis: simultaneous determination of 5-hydroxytryptophol glucuronide and 5-hydroxyindoleacetic acid by direct injection of urine using ultra-performance liquid chromatography-tandem mass spectrometry. J Mass Spect 2007;42: 940-949.

CPT Code:
Column chromatography/ mass spectrometry: quantitative, single stationary and mobile phase 82542

INSULIN

Reference Interval

4–24 µU/mL

Procedure

Insulin is measured by direct radioimmunoassay.

Patient Preparation

The patient should fast for 10 to 12 hours prior to collection of specimen. The patient should not take any medications that influence insulin production or secretion, if possible, for at least 48 hours prior to collection of specimen.

Specimen Collection

Collect 3mL serum and separate as soon as possible. Freeze serum immediately after separation. Minimum specimen size is 1mL.

Special Specimens

For special fluids, such as CSF, vitreous fluid, peritoneal fluid, synovial fluid, contact ISI for requirements and special handling instructions.

Shipping Instructions

Ship specimens frozen in dry ice.

References
1. Wild RA, Applebaum-Bowden D, Demers LM, et alJ. Lipoprotein lipids in women with androgen excess: independent associations with increased insulin and androgen. Clin Chem (Oxf). 1990; 36:283-9.
2. Argoud GM, Schad DS, Eaton RP. Insulin suppresses its own secretion in vivo. Diabetes. 1987;36:959-62.
3. Chevenne D, Trivin F, Porquet D. Insulin assays and reference values. Diabetes Metab. 1999;25(6):459-76.

CPT Code:
Insulin 83525

INTERLEUKINS 1-18 (IL 1-18)

Reference Interval

Reference range is listed on individual patient test reports. Interleukins available include: IL-1α, IL-1β, IL-2, IL-3, IL-4, IL-5, II-6, IL-7, IL-8, IL-10, IL-12, IL-13, IL-18.

Procedure

The Interleukin assays are measured by direct radioimmunoassay/enzyme immunoassay.

Patient Preparation

The patient should not be on any corticosteroids, anti-inflammatory medications or pain killers, if possible, for at least 48 hours prior to collection of specimen.

Specimen Collection

Collect 3mL serum or EDTA plasma and separate as soon as possible. Freeze serum or plasma immediately after separation. Minimum specimen size is 1mL.

Special Specimens

For special fluids, such as CSF, vitreous fluid, peritoneal fluid, synovial fluid, contact ISI for requirements and special handling instructions.

Shipping Instructions

Ship specimens frozen in dry ice.

References
1. Lieb DC, Parson HK, Mamikunian G, Vinik Al. Cardiac autonomic imbalance in newly diagnosed and established diabetes is associated with markers of adipose tissue inflammation. Exp Diabetes Res. Research Article. 2012;2012:878760.Epub.2011 Nov 1.
2. Ward WK, Paquette TL, Frank BH, et al. A sensitive radioimmunoassay for human proinsulin with sequential use of antisera to peptide and insulin. Clin Chem (Oxf). 1986;32:728-33.
3. Shetty MR, Boghossian HM, Duffell D, et al. Tumor-induced hypoglycemia: a result of ectopic insulin production. Cancer. 1982;May;49(9):1920-3.
4. Rutter GA. Insulin secretion: feed-forward control of insulin biosynthesis? Curr Biol. 1999;9(12):R443-4.
5. Sapin R. Insulin assays: previously known and new analytical features. Clin Lab. 2003;49(3-4):113-21.
6. Jia EZ, Yang ZJ, Chen SW, Qi GY, You CF, Ma JF, Zhang JX, Wang ZZ, Qian WC, Li XL, Wang HY, Ma WZ. Significant association of insulin and proinsulin with clustering of cardiovascular risk factors. World J Gastroenterol. 2005;11(1):149-53.
7. Pfutzner A, Pfutzner AH, Larbig M, Forst T. Role of intact proinsulin in diagnosis and treatment of type 2 diabetes mellitus. Diabetes Technol Ther. 2004;6(3):405-12.
8. Wiesli P, Perren A, Saremaslani P, Pfammatter T, Spinas GA, Schmid C. Abnormalities of proinsulin processing in functioning insulinomas: clinical implications. Clin Endocrinol (Oxf). 2004;61(4):424-30.
9. Gama R, Teale JD, Marks V. Best practice No 173: clinical and laboratory investigation of adult spontaneous hypoglycaemia. J Clin Pathol. 2003;56(9):641-6.
10. Pozzilli P, Manfrini S, Monetini L. Biochemical markers of type 1 diabetes: clinical use. Scand J Clin Lab Invest (Suppl). 2001;235:38-44.

CPT Code:
Unspecified Quantitative Immunoassay 83519

LANREOTIDE (SOMATULINE® DEPOT)

Reference Interval

Lanreotide administered as Somatuline® Depot
480 mg/month: 20,000 pg/mL ± 2,000 pg/mL
240 mg/month: 10,000 pg/mL ± 2,000 pg/mL
120 mg/month: 5,000 pg/mL ± 1,000 pg/mL
90 mg/month: 2,500 pg/mL ± 500 pg/mL

Procedure

Lanreotide is measured by direct radioimmunoassay.

Patient Preparation

This test is only useful for those patients being treated with Lanreotide. No special preparation is necessary since Lanreotide is not a naturally occurring substance. For optimal results, specimen should be collected immediately before the next injection of Lanreotide (trough levels) and after having been on the medication at least four months. Additional Lanreotide levels should be drawn in patients with evidence of tumor progression or loss of symptom control.

Specimen Collection

Collect 3mL serum or EDTA plasma and separate as soon as possible. Specimen is stable room temperature three days; refrigerated one week and frozen for several years. Minimum specimen size is 1mL.

Special Specimens

For special fluids, such as CSF, vitreous fluid, peritoneal fluid, synovial fluid, contact ISI for requirements and special handling instructions.

Shipping Instructions

Ship specimens ambient, refrigerated, or frozen in dry ice.

Reference
  1. Personal data generated by E.A. Woltering, M.D. unpublished data.

CPT Code:
Therapeutic Drug Assay: Quantitation of Drug, Not Elsewhere Specified 80299

LEPTIN

Reference Interval

Reference range is listed on individual patient test reports.

Procedure

Leptin is measured by direct radioimmunoassay.

Patient Preparation

The patient should fast for 10 to 12 hours prior to collection of specimen. The patient should not take any medications that influence insulin production or secretion, if possible.

Specimen Collection

Collect 10mL blood directly into ISI's G.I. Preservative tube and separate as soon as possible. Freeze plasma immediately after separation. Special G.I. Preservative tubes are available from ISI. Minimum specimen size is 1mL.

Important Precaution

Leptin specimens must be collected using ISI's G.I. Preservative tube. No other methods of collection are acceptable.

Special Specimens

For special fluids, such as CSF, vitreous fluid, peritoneal fluid, synovial fluid, contact ISI for requirements and special handling instructions.

Shipping Instructions

Ship specimens frozen in dry ice.

References
1. Lieb DC, Parson HK, Mamikunian G, Vinik AI. Cardiac autonomic imbalance in newly diagnosed and established diabetes is associated with markers of adipose tissue inflammation. Exp Diabetes Res. Research Article. 2012;2012:878760.Epub.2011 Nov 1.
2. Valle M, Martos R, Gascon F, et al. Low-grade systemic inflammation, hypoadiponectinemia and a high concentration of leptin are present in very young obese children, and correlate with metabolic syndrome. Diabetes Metab. 2005;Feb;31(1):55-62.
3. Er H, Doganay S, Ozerol E, et al. Adrenomedullin and leptin levels in diabetic retinopathy and retinal diseases. Ophthalmologica. 2005;Mar-Apr;219(2):107-11.
4. Mars M, de Graaf C, de Groot LC, et al. Decreases in fasting leptin and insulin concentrations after acute energy restriction and subsequent compensation in food intake. Am J Clin Nutr. 2005;Mar;81(3):570-7.
5. Abdella NA, Mojiminiyi OA, Moussa MA, Zaki M, Al Mohammedi H, Al Ozairi ES, Al Jebely S. Plasma leptin concentration in patients with Type 2 diabetes: relationship to cardiovascular disease risk factors and insulin resistance. Diabet Med. 2005;Mar;22(3):278-85.
6. Boden G, Sargrad K, Homko C, Mozzoli M, Stein TP. Effect of a low-carbohydrate diet on appetite, blood glucose levels, and insulin resistance in obese patients with type 2 diabetes. Ann Intern Med. 2005;15 Mar;142(6):403-11.

CPT Code:
Unspecified Quantitative Immunoassay 83519

MELANOCYTE STIMULATING HORMONE, ALPHA (α-MSH)

Reference Interval

Up to 5.0 pg/mL

Procedure

Alpha-MSH is measured by direct radioimmunoassay.

Patient Preparation

The patient should not be on any steroid, ACTH or hypertension medication, if possible, for at least 48 hours prior to collection of specimen. Morning, fasting specimens are preferred; however, non-fasting specimens are acceptable.

Specimen Collection

Collect 3mL serum or EDTA plasma and separate as soon as possible. Freeze serum or plasma immediately after separation. Minimum specimen size is 1mL.

Special Specimens

For special fluids, such as CSF, vitreous fluid, peritoneal fluid, synovial fluid, contact ISI for requirements and special handling instructions.

Shipping Instructions

Ship specimens frozen in dry ice.

References
1. Seifer DB and Collins RL. Current concepts of endorphin physiology in female reproductive dysfunction. Clin Chem. 1990;54:757-771.
2. Shapiro M, Nicholson WE, Orth DN, Mitchell WM, Lidddle GW. Differences between ectopic MSH and pituitary MSH. J Clin Endocrinol Metab. 1971;33:377-381.

CPT Code:
Unspecified Quantitative Immunoassay 83519

MELANOCYTE STIMULATING HORMONE, BETA (β-MSH)

Reference Interval

Up to 150 pg/mL

Procedure

Beta-MSH is measured by direct radioimmunoassay.

Patient Preparation

The patient should not be on any steroid, ACTH or hypertension medication, if possible, for at least 48 hours prior to collection of specimen. Morning, fasting specimens are preferred; however, non-fasting specimens are acceptable.

Specimen Collection

Collect 3mL serum or EDTA plasma and separate as soon as possible. Freeze serum or plasma immediately after separation. Minimum specimen size is 1mL.

Special Specimens

For special fluids, such as CSF, vitreous fluid, peritoneal fluid, synovial fluid, contact ISI for requirements and special handling instructions.

Shipping Instructions

Ship specimens frozen in dry ice.

References
1. Seifer DB and Collins RL. Current concepts of endorphin physiology in female reproductive dysfunction. Clin Chem. 1990;54:757-771.
2. Shapiro M, Nicholson WE, Orth DN, Mitchell WM, Lidddle GW. Differences between ectopic MSH and pituitary MSH. J Clin Endocrinol Metab. 1971;33:377-381.

CPT Code:
Unspecified Quantitative Immunoassay 83519

MELANOCYTE STIMULATING HORMONE, GAMMA (γ-MSH)

Reference Interval

Up to 150 pg/mL

Procedure

Gamma-MSH is measured by direct radioimmunoassay.

Patient Preparation

The patient should not be on any steroid, ACTH or hypertension medication, if possible, for at least 48 hours prior to collection of specimen. Morning, fasting specimens are preferred; however, non-fasting specimens are acceptable.

Specimen Collection

Collect 3mL serum or EDTA plasma and separate as soon as possible. Freeze serum or plasma immediately after separation. Minimum specimen size is 1mL.

Special Specimens

For special fluids, such as CSF, vitreous fluid, peritoneal fluid, synovial fluid, contact ISI for requirements and special handling instructions.

Shipping Instructions

Ship specimens frozen in dry ice.

References
1. Seifer DB and Collins RL. Current concepts of endorphin physiology in female reproductive dysfunction. Clin Chem. 1990;54:757-771.
2. Nakai Y, Tanaka I, Fukata J, Nakao K, Oki S, Takai S, Imura H. Evidence for γ-MSH-like immunoreacativity in ectopic ACTH-producing tumors. J Clin Endocrinol Metab. 1980;50:1147-1148.

CPT Code:
Unspecified Quantitative Immunoassay 83519

MELATONIN

Reference Interval

Up to 8 pg/mL (Daylight or bright levels). See report for pediatric and dark cycle levels.

Procedure

Melatonin is measured by direct radioimmunoassay.

Patient Preparation

For dark cycle baseline collections inpatients should be drawn during the nighttime, dark cycle (2AM-4AM) and should not be exposed to bright light during the collection period. Patients should not be on any steroid, ACTH or Gonadotropin medications, if possible, for at least 48 hours prior to collection of specimen.

Specimen Collection

Collect 3mL EDTA serum or plasma and separate as soon as possible. Freeze serum or plasma immediately after separation. Minimum specimen size is 1mL.

Special Specimens

For special fluids, such as CSF, vitreous fluid, peritoneal fluid, synovial fluid, contact ISI for requirements and special handling instructions.

Shipping Instructions

Ship specimens frozen in dry ice.

References
1. Sack RL, Lewy AJ. Melatonin and major affective disorders in melatonin: clinical perspectives. eds Miles A, Philbrick DRS, and Thompson C. Oxford Med Pub 1988, 205-227.
2. Arendt J, Panier L and Sizonenko PC. Melatonin radioimmunoassay. J Clin Endocrinol Metab. 1975, 40:347.
3 Leon J, Acuña-Castroviejo D, Sainz RM, Mayo JC, Tan DX, Reiter RJ. Melatonin and mitochondrial function. Life Sci. 2004;75:765-90.

CPT Code:
Unspecified Quantitative Immunoassay 83519

MOTILIN

Reference Interval

Up to 446 pg/mL

Procedure

Motilin is measured by direct radioimmunoassay.

Patient Preparation

The patient should fast for 10 to 12 hours prior to collection of specimen. Antacid medications and medications that affect intestinal motility should be discontinued, if possible, for at least 48 hours prior to collection of specimen.

Specimen Collection

Collect 3mL serum or EDTA plasma and separate as soon as possible. Freeze serum or plasma immediately after separation. Minimum specimen size is 1mL.

Special Specimens

For special fluids, such as CSF, vitreous fluid, peritoneal fluid, synovial fluid, contact ISI for requirements and special handling instructions.

Shipping Instructions

Ship specimens frozen in dry ice.

References
1. Dea D, Boileau G, Poitras P, et al. Molecular heterogeneity of human motilin like immunoreactivity explained by the processing of prepromotilin. Gastroenterology. 1989;Mar;96(3):695-703.

CPT Code:
Unspecified Quantitative Immunoassay 83519

NEUROKININ A (NKA; SUBSTANCE K)

Reference Interval

Up to 40 pg/mL

Procedure

NKA is measured by direct radioimmunoassay.

Patient Preparation

The patient should not take pain relievers or any medications that affect hypertension or gastrointestinal function, if possible, for at least 48 hours prior to collection of specimen.

Specimen Collection

Collect 10mL blood directly into ISI's Z-tube™ Preservative and separate as soon as possible. Freeze plasma immediately after separation. Special Z-tube™ Preservatives are available from ISI. Minimum specimen size is 1mL.

Important Precaution

NKA plasma specimens must be collected using ISI's Z-tube™ Preservative. No other methods of collection are acceptable.

Special Specimens

*Frozen Z-tube™ plasma is the only acceptable sample type for this assay.

Shipping Instructions

Ship specimens frozen in dry ice.

References
1. Mamikunian P, Ardill JES, O'Dorisio TM, et al.Validation of neurokinin A (NKA) assays in the United States and Europe. Pancreas. 2011;40(7).1000-5.
2. Diebold AE, Boudreaux JP, Wang YZ et al. Neurokinin A levels predict survival in patients with well differentiated small bowel neuroendocrine tumors. Surgery. In Press.
3. Kimuro S, Okada M, Sugata Y. Novel neuropeptides neurokinin alpha and beta, isolated from porcine spinal cord. Proc Japan Acad. 1983;59:101.
4. Nawa H, Kotani H, Nakanishi S. Tissue specific generation of tissue pre-pro-tachykinin mRNAs from one gene by alternative RNA splicing. Nature. 1984-5;312(5996):729-34.
5. Theodorsson-Norheim E, Norheim I, et alG. Neuropeptide K: a major tachykinin in plasma and tumor tissues from carcinoid patients. Biochem Biophys Res Commun. 1985;131(1):77-83.
6. Conlon JM, Deacon CF, Richter G, et al. Measurement and partial characterization of the multiple forms of neurokinin A-like immunoreactivity in carcinoid tumours. Regul Pept. 1986;Jan;13(2):183-96.
7. Hunt RH, Tougas G. Evolving concepts in functional gastrointestinal disorders: promising directions for novel pharmaceutical treatments. Best Pract Res Clin Gastroenterol. 2002;16(6):869-83.
8. Ardill JE, Erikkson B. The importance of the measurement of circulating markers in patients with neuroendocrine tumours of the pancreas and gut. Endocr Relat Cancer. 2003;10(4):459-62.
9. Chen LW, Yung KK, Chan YS. Neurokinin peptides and neurokinin receptors as potential therapeutic intervention targets of basal ganglia in the prevention and treatment of Parkinson's disease. Curr Drug Targets. 2004;5(2):197-206.
10. Severini C, Ciotti MT, Mercanti D, et al. The tachykinin peptide family. Pharmacol Rev.2002;54(2):285-322.
11. Pennefather JN, Lecci A, Candenas ML, et al. Tachykinins and tachykinin receptors: a growing family. Life Sci. 2004;74(12):1445-63.

CPT Code:
Unspecified Quantitative Immunoassay 83519

NEUROPEPTIDE Y (NPY)

Reference Interval

154 - 513 pg/mL

Procedure

NPY is measured by direct radioimmunoassay.

Patient Preparation

The patient should fast for 10 to 12 hours prior to collection of specimen. Medications that affect insulin secretion or gastrointestinal function should be discontinued, if possible, for at least 48 hours prior to collection of specimen.

Specimen Collection

Collect 10mL blood directly into ISI's Z-tube™ Preservative and separate as soon as possible. Freeze plasma immediately after separation. Special Z-tube™ Preservatives are available from ISI. Minimum specimen size is 1mL.

Important Precaution

NPY plasma specimens must be collected using ISI's Z-tube™ Preservative. No other methods of collection are acceptable.

Special Specimens

*Frozen Z-tube™ plasma is the only acceptable sample type for this assay.

Shipping Instructions

Ship specimens frozen in dry ice.

References
1. Jamal H, Jones PM, Byrne J, et al. Peptide contents of neuropeptide Y, vasoactive intestinal polypeptide, and β-calcitonin gene-related peptide and their messenger ribonucleic acids after dexamethasone treatment in the isolated rat islets of langerhans. Endocrinology. 1991;129:3372-80.
2. Lehmann J. Neuropeptide Y: an overview. Drug Dev Res. 1989; 19:329-51.
3. O'Dorisio MS, Hauger M, O'Dorisio TM. Age-dependent levels of plasma neuropeptides in normal children. Regul Pept. 2002;109(1-3):189-92.
4. Gehlert DR. Introduction to the reviews on neuropeptide Y. Neuropeptides. 2004;38(4):135-40.
5. Zoccali C. Neuropeptide Y as a far-reaching neuromediator: from energy balance and cardiovascular regulation to central integration of weight and bone mass control mechanisms. Implications for human diseases. Curr Opin Nephrol Hypertens.2005;14(1):25-32.
6. Beaujouan JC, Torrens Y, Saffroy M, et al. A 25 year adventure in the field of tachykinins. Peptides. 2004;25(3):339-57.
7. Oberg K. Biochemical diagnosis of neuroendocrine GEP tumor. Yale J Biol Med. 1997;70(5-6):501-8.
8. Makridis C, Theodorsson E, Akerstrom G, et al. Increased intestinal non-substance P tachykinin concentrations in malignant midgut carcinoid disease. J Gastroenterol Hepatol. 1999;14(5):500-7.

CPT Code:
Unspecified Quantitative Immunoassay 83519

NEUROTENSIN

Reference Interval

50–100 pg/mL

Procedure

Neurotensin is measured by direct radioimmunoassay.

Patient Preparation

The patient should fast for 10 to 12 hours prior to collection of specimen. Antacid medications and medications that affect gastrointestinal function should be discontinued, if possible, for at least 48 hours prior to collection of specimen.

Specimen Collection

Collect 10mL blood directly into ISI's Z-tube™ Preservative and separate as soon as possible. Freeze plasma immediately after separation. Special Z-tube™ Preservatives are available from ISI. Minimum specimen size is 1mL.

Important Precaution

Neurotensin plasma specimens must be collected using ISI's Z-tube™ Preservative. No other methods of collection are acceptable.

Special Specimens

*Frozen Z-tube™ plasma is the only acceptable sample type for this assay.

Shipping Instructions

Ship specimens frozen in dry ice.

References
1. Shulkes A, Chick P, Wong H, et al. A radioimmunoassay for neurotensin in human plasma. Clin Chim Acta. 13 1982;Oct;125(1):49-58.
2. Carraway RE, Mitra SP, Feurle GE, et al. Presence of neurotensin and neuromedin-N within a common precursor from a human pancreatic neuroendocrine tumor. J Clin Endocrinol Metab. 1988;Jun;66(6):1323-8.
3. Reubi JC. Peptide receptors as molecular targets for cancer diagnosis and therapy. Endocr Rev. 2003;24(4):389-427.

CPT Code:
Unspecified Quantitative Immunoassay 83519

OCTREOTIDE (SANDOSTATIN®)

Reference Intervals for Therapeutic Octreotide Levels

Long-acting repeatable (LAR) dose-response levels: mean octreotide level ± 2 SD for patients on octreotide LAR for 3 or more months (steady-state). The following represent trough levels measured immediately before an injection of LAR.

Octreotide administered by pump:
60 mg/month: 10,000 pg/mL ± 2,500 pg/mL
30 mg/month: 5,000 pg/mL ± 2,500 pg/mL

Octreotide administered as Sandostatin® LAR:
120 mg/month: 9,000 pg/mL ± 2,000 pg/mL
60 mg/month: 5,000 pg/mL ± 2,000 pg/mL
30 mg/month: 2,500 pg/mL ± 1,500 pg/mL

Octreotide administered by subcutaneous injection:
Measurement of plasma octreotide is not recommended for individuals using multiple daily octreotide injections due to the short half life of octreotide in the plasma (approximately 90–120 minutes).

Procedure

Octreotide is measured by direct radioimmunoassay. There is no cross-reactivity with native somatostatin-14 or somatostatin-28. There also is no cross-reactivity with Lanreotide; therefore, this test should not be used to measure blood levels of this drug.

Patient Preparation

This test is useful only for those patients being treated with octreotide acetate. No special preparation is needed for this test. For optimal results, blood for this test should be drawn immediately before the patient's next injection of octreotide LAR (trough levels). Fasting is not required. Octreotide levels are not recommended for patients taking multiple, daily sub-cutaneous injections of Octreotide to guide therapy. However, patients receiving continuous subcutaneous infusion of Octreotide by pump can measure blood levels anytime while the pump is running. Levels may vary weight and sex. Additional lanreotide levels should be drawn in patients with evidence of tumor progression or loss of symptom control.

Specimen Collection

Collect 3mL serum or EDTA plasma and separate as soon as possible. Octreotide is stable at room temperature for 3 days. Specimens can be stored room temperature, refrigerated, or frozen in dry ice. Minimum specimen size is 1mL.

Special Specimens

For special fluids, such as CSF, vitreous fluid, peritoneal fluid, synovial fluid, contact ISI for requirements and special handling instructions.

Shipping Instructions

Ship specimens ambient, refrigerated, or frozen in dry ice.

CPT Code:
Therapeutic Drug Assay: Quantitation of Drug, Not Elsewhere Specified 80299

References
1. Anthony L, Vinik AI. Evaluating the characteristics and the management of patients with neuroendocrine tumors receiving octreotide LAR during a 6-year period. Pancreas.2011;40:987-94.
2. Woltering EA, Mamikunian PM, Zietz S, et al. The effect of octreotide LAR dose and weight on octreotide blood levels in patients with neuroendocrine tumors. Pancreas. 2005;31(4):392-400.
3. Woltering EA, Salvo VA, O'Dorisio TM, et al. Clinical value of monitoring plasma octreotide levels during chronic octreotide long-acting repeatable therapy in carcinoid patients. Pancreas. 2008;Jul;37(1):94-100.
4. Woltering EA, Hilton RS, Zolfoghary CM, et al. Validation of serum versus plasma measurements of chromogranin a levels in patients with carcinoid tumors: lack of correlation between absolute chromogranin a levels and symptom frequency. Pancreas. 2006;Oct;33(3):250-4.

PANCREASTATIN

Reference Interval

10–135 pg/mL

Procedure

Pancreastatin is measured by direct radioimmunoassay.

Patient Preparation

The patient should fast for 10 to 12 hours prior to collection of specimen. The patient should not take any medications that influence insulin levels, if possible, for at least 48 hours prior to collection of specimen.

Specimen Collection

Collect 10mL blood directly into ISI's Z-tube™ Preservative and separate as soon as possible. Freeze plasma immediately after separation. Special Z-tube™ Preservatives are available from ISI. Minimum specimen size is 1mL.

Important Precaution

Pancreastatin plasma specimens must be collected using ISI's Z-tube™ Preservative. No other methods of collection are acceptable.

Special Specimens

*Frozen Z-tube™ plasma is the only acceptable sample type for this assay.

Shipping Instructions

Ship specimens frozen in dry ice.

References
1. Raines D, Chester M, Diebold AE, et al. A prospective evaluation of the effect of chronic proton pump inhibitor use on plasma biomarker levels in humans. Pancreas. 2012;41(4):508-511.
2. O'Dorisio TM, Krutzik SR, Woltering EA, et al. Development of a highly sensitive and specific carboxy-terminal human Pancreastatin assay to monitor neuroendocrine tumor behavior. Pancreas. 2010;39(5):611-616.
3. Piero E, Mirelles P, Silvestre RA, et al. Pancreastatin inhibits insulin secretion as induced by glucagon, vasoactive intestinal polypeptide, gastric inhibiting peptide, and 8-cholecystokinin in the perfused rat pancreas. Metabolism. 1989;38:679-82.
4. Tatemoto K, Efendi S, Mutt S, et al. Pancreastatin, a novel pancreatic peptide that inhibits insulin secretion. Nature. 1986;324:476-8.
5. Calhoun K, Toth-Fejel S, Chee J, et al. Serum peptide profiles in patients with carcinoid tumors. Am J Surg. 2003;186(1):28-31.
6. Syversen U, Jacobsen MB, O'Connor DT, et al. Immunoassays for measurement of chromogranin A and pancreastatin-like immunoreactivity in humans: correspondence in patients with neuroendocrine neoplasia. Neuropeptides. 1994;26(3):201-6.
7. Kogner P, Bjellerup P, Svensson T, et al. Pancreastatin immunoreactivity in favourable childhood neuroblastoma and ganglioneuroma. Eur J Cancer 1995;31A(4):557-60.
8. Desai DC, O'Dorisio TM, Schirmer WJ, et al. Serum pancreastatin levels predict response to hepatic artery chemoembolization and somatostatin analog therapy in metastatic neuroendocrine tumors. Regul Pept. 2001;96(3):113-17.

CPT Code:
Unspecified Quantitative Immunoassay 83519

PANCREATIC POLYPEPTIDE (PP)

Reference Interval (Fasting)

Age (year)	Range (pg/mL)
20–29	10–140
30–39	20–500
40–49	25–880
50–59	25–925
60–69	40–600

Procedure

PP is measured by direct radioimmunoassay.

Patient Preparation

The patient should fast for 10 to 12 hours prior to collection of specimen. Antacid medications and medications that affect insulin levels should be discontinued, if possible, for at least 48 hours prior to collection of specimen. Diabetes and gastric procedures can affect the fasting levels.

Specimen Collection

Collect 3mL serum or EDTA plasma and separate as soon as possible. Freeze serum or plasma immediately after separation. Minimum specimen size is 1mL.

Special Specimens

For special fluids, such as CSF, vitreous fluid, peritoneal fluid, synovial fluid, contact ISI for requirements and special handling instructions.

Shipping Instructions

Ship specimens frozen in dry ice.

References

1. Kennedy FP, Go VLW, Cryer PE, et al. Subnormal pancreatic polypeptide and epinephrine response to insulin-induced hypoglycemia identify patients with insulin-dependent diabetes mellitus predisposal to develop overt autonomic neuropathy. Ann Intern Med. 1988.;Jan;108(1):54-8.
2. Stern AI, Hansky J. Pancreatic polypeptide release in gastric ulcer. Dig Dis Sci. 1981; Apr;26(4):289-91.
3. Druce MR, Small CJ, Bloom SR. Minireview: gut peptides regulating satiety. Endocrinology. 2004;145(6):2660-5.
4. Small CJ, Bloom SR. Gut hormones and the control of appetite. Trends Endocrinol Metab. 2004;15(6):259-63.
5. Batterham RL, Le Roux CW, Cohen MA, et al. Pancreatic polypeptide reduces appetite and food intake in humans. J Clin Endocrinol Metab. 2003;88(8):3989-92.
6. Panzuto F, Severi C, Cannizzaro R, et al. Utility of combined use of plasma levels of chromogranin A and pancreatic polypeptide in the diagnosis of gastrointestinal and pancreatic endocrine tumors. J Endocrinol Invest. 2004;27(1):6-11.
7. Yamashita Y, Miyahara E, Shimizu K, et al. Screening of gastrointestinal hormone release in patients with lung cancer. In Vivo.2003;17(2):193-5.

CPT Code:
Unspecified Quantitative Immunoassay 83519

PEPSINOGEN I (PG I)

Reference Interval

28–100 ng/mL

Procedure

PG I is measured by direct radioimmunoassay.

Patient Preparation

The patient should fast for 10 to 12 hours prior to collection of specimen. Antacid medications or medications that affect intestinal motility should be discontinued, if possible, for at least 48 hours prior to collection of specimen.

Specimen Collection

Collect 3mL serum or EDTA plasma and separate as soon as possible. Freeze serum or plasma immediately after separation. Minimum specimen size is 1mL.

Special Specimens

For special fluids, such as CSF, vitreous fluid, peritoneal fluid, synovial fluid, contact ISI for requirements and special handling instructions.

Shipping Instructions

Ship specimens frozen in dry ice.

References
1. Plebani M, DiMario F, Dal Santo PL, et al. Measurement of pepsinogen group I in endoscopic gastroduodenal biopsies. Clin Chem. 1990;36:682-4.
2. Samloff IM, Liebman WM. Radioimmunoassay of group I pepsinogens in serum. Gastroenterology. 1974;Apr;66(4):494-502.

CPT Code:
Unspecified Quantitative Immunoassay 83519

PEPSINOGEN II (PG II)

Reference Interval

Up to 22 ng/mL

Procedure

PG II is measured by direct radioimmunoassay.

Patient Preparation

The patient should fast for 10 to 12 hours prior to collection of specimen. Antacid medications or medications that affect intestinal motility should be discontinued, if possible, for at least 48 hours prior to collection of specimen.

Specimen Collection

Collect 3mL serum or EDTA plasma and separate as soon as possible. Freeze serum or plasma immediately after separation. Minimum specimen size is 1mL.

Special Specimens

For special fluids, such as CSF, vitreous fluid, peritoneal fluid, synovial fluid, contact ISI for requirements and special handling instructions.

Shipping Instructions

Ship specimens frozen in dry ice.

References
1. Plebani M, Masiero M, DiMario F, et al. Radioimmunoassay for pepsinogen C. Clin Chem. 1990;36(9):1690.
2. Matzku S, Zoller M, Rapp W. Radioimmunological quantification of human group-II pepsinogens. Digestion. 1978;18(1-2):16-26.

CPT Code:
Unspecified Quantitative Immunoassay 83519

PEPTIDE HISTIDINE ISOLEUCINE (PHIM)

Reference Interval

10–40 pg/mL

Procedure

PHIM is measured by direct radioimmunoassay.

Patient Preparation

The patient should fast for 10 to 12 hours prior to collection of specimen. Antacid medications and medications that affect intestinal motility should be discontinued, if possible, for at least 48 hours prior to collection of specimen.

Specimen Collection

Collect 10mL blood directly into ISI's G.I. Preservative tube and separate as soon as possible. Freeze plasma immediately after separation. Special G.I. Preservative tubes are available from ISI. Minimum specimen size is 1mL.

Important Precaution

PHIM specimens must be collected using ISI's G.I. Preservative tube. No other methods of collection are acceptable.

Special Specimens

For special fluids, such as CSF, vitreous fluid, peritoneal fluid, synovial fluid, contact ISI for requirements and special handling instructions.

Shipping Instructions

Ship specimens frozen in dry ice.

References
1. Lieb DC, Parson HK, Mamikunian G, Vinik AI. Cardiac autonomic imbalance in newly diagnosed and established diabetes is associated with markers of adipose tissue inflammation. Exp Diabetes Res. Research Article 2012;2012:878760.Epub.2011 Nov 1.
2. Yiango Y, Christofides ND, Blank MA, et al. Molecular forms of peptide histidine isoleucine-like immunoreactivity in the gastrointestinal tract. Gastroenterology. 1985;Sep;89(3):516-24.
3. Christofides ND, Yiangou Y, Aarons E. Radioimmunoassay and intramural distribution of PHI-IR in the human intestine. DigDis Sci. 1983;Jun;28(6):507-12.
4. Fahrenkrug J, Hannibal J. Neurotransmitters co-existing with VIP or PACAP. Peptides. 2004;25(3):393-401.
5. D'Souza M, Plevak D, Kvols L, Shine T, Stapelfeldt W, Nelson D, Southorn P, Murray M. Elevated neuropeptide levels decrease during liver transplant. Transplant Proc. 1993;25(2):1805-6.

CPT Code:
Unspecified Quantitative Immunoassay 83519

PEPTIDE YY (PYY)

Reference Interval

30–120 pg/mL

Procedure

PYY is measured by direct radioimmunoassay.

Patient Preparation

The patient should fast for 10 to 12 hours prior to collection of specimen. Antacid medications and medications that affect intestinal motility should be discontinued, if possible, for at least 48 hours prior to collection of specimen.

Specimen Collection

Collect 10mL blood directly into ISI's G.I. Preservative tube and separate as soon as possible. Freeze plasma immediately after separation. Special G.I. Preservative tubes are available from ISI. Minimum specimen size is 1mL.

Important Precaution

PYY specimens must be collected using ISI's G.I. Preservative tube. No other methods of collection are acceptable.

Special Specimens

For special fluids, such as CSF, vitreous fluid, peritoneal fluid, synovial fluid, contact ISI for requirements and special handling instructions.

Shipping Instructions

Ship specimens frozen in dry ice.

References
1. Adrian TE, Ferri GL, Bacarese-Hamilton AJ, et al. Human distribution and release of a putative new gut hormone, peptide YY. Gastroenterology.1985;Nov;89(5):1070-7.
2. Adrian TE, Bacarese-Hamilton AJ, Savage AP, et al. Peptide YY abnormalities in gastrointestinal diseases. Gastroenterology. 1986;Feb;90(2):379-84.
3. Lin HC, Chey WY. Cholecystokinin and peptide YY are released by fat in either proximal or distal small intestine in dogs. Regul Pept.2003;114(2-3):131-5.
4. McGowan BM, Bloom SR. Peptide YY and appetite control. Curr Opin Pharmacol.2004;4(6):583-8.

CPT Code:
Unspecified Quantitative Immunoassay 83519

PLASMINOGEN ACTIVATOR INHIBITOR 1 (PAI-1)

Reference Interval

Up to 1.0 IU/mL

Procedure

PAI-1 is measured by direct radioimmunoassay.

Patient Preparation

The patient should fast for 10 to 12 hours prior to collection of specimen. Antacid medications and medications that affect intestinal motility should be discontinued, if possible, for at least 48 hours prior to collection of specimen.

Specimen Collection

Collect 10mL blood directly into ISI's G.I. Preservative tube and separate as soon as possible. Freeze plasma immediately after separation. Special G.I. Preservative tubes are available from ISI. Minimum specimen size is 1mL.

Important Precaution

PAI-1 specimens must be collected using ISI's G.I. Preservative tube. No other methods of collection are acceptable.

Special Specimens

For special fluids, such as CSF, vitreous fluid, peritoneal fluid, synovial fluid, contact ISI for requirements and special handling instructions.

Shipping Instructions

Ship specimens frozen in dry ice.

References
1. Lieb DC, Parson HK, Mamikunian G, Vinik AI. Cardiac autonomic imbalance in newly diagnosed and established diabetes is associated with markers of adipose tissue inflammation. Exp Diabetes Res. Research Article. 2012;2012:878760.Epub.2011 Nov 1.
2. Juhan-Vague I, Alessi MC, Vague P. Increased plasma plasminogen activator inhibitor I levels. A possible link between insulin resistance and atherothrombosis. Diabetologia.1991;34:457-62.
3. Landin K, Tengborn L, Smith U. Elevated fibrinogen and plasminogen activator inhibitor (PAI-I) in hypertension are related to metabolic risk factors for cardiovascular disease. J Intern Med.1990;227:273-8.

CPT Code:
PAI-1 85420–85421

PROSTAGLANDIN D2 (PG D2)

Reference Interval

35–115 pg/mL

Procedure

PG D2 is measured by radioimmunoassay/EIA/ELISA following extraction of specimens.

Patient Preparation

The patient should not take aspirin, indomethacin, or anti-inflammatory medications, if possible, for at least 48 hours prior to collection of specimen.

Specimen Collection

Collect 3mL serum or EDTA plasma and separate as soon as possible. Freeze serum or plasma immediately after separation. Minimum specimen size is 1mL.

Special Specimens

For special fluids, such as CSF, vitreous fluid, peritoneal fluid, synovial fluid, contact ISI for requirements and special handling instructions.

Shipping Instructions

Ship specimens frozen in dry ice.

References
1. Redfern JS, Feldman M. Role of endogenous prostaglandins in preventing gastrointestinal ulceration: induction of ulcers by antibodies to prostaglandins. Gastroenterology.1989;Feb;96(2 Pt 2 Suppl):596-605.
2. Bennegard B, Hahlin M, Hamberger L. Luteotropic effects of prostaglandins I2 and D2 on isolated human corpora luteum. Fertil Steril. 1990;Sep;54(3):459-64.

CPT Code:
Prostaglandin D2 84150

PROSTAGLANDIN D2 (PG D2), URINE

Reference Interval

100–280 ng/24 hours

Procedure

PG D2 is measured by direct radioimmunoassay/EIA/ELISA.

Patient Preparation

The patient should not take aspirin, indomethacin, or anti-inflammatory medications, if possible, for at least 48 hours prior to collection of specimen.

Specimen Collection

Submit 5mL of a well mixed 24-hour urine collection. No special preservatives are required. Minimum specimen size is 1mL. Provide total volume per 24 hours, if possible; however, random urine samples are acceptable.

Shipping Instructions

Ship specimens frozen in dry ice.

References
1. Redfern JS, Feldman M. Role of endogenous prostaglandins in preventing gastrointestinal ulceration: induction of ulcers by antibodies to prostaglandins. Gastroenterology.1989;Feb;96(2 Pt 2 Suppl):596-605.
2. Bennegard B, Hahlin M, Hamberger L. Luteotropic effects of prostaglandins I2 and D2 on isolated human corpora luteum. Fertil Steril.1990;Sep;54(3):459-64.

CPT Code:
Prostaglandin D2 84150

PROSTAGLANDIN E1 (PG E1)

Reference Interval

250–500 pg/mL

Procedure

PG E1 is measured by radioimmunoassay/EIA/ELISA following extraction of specimens.

Patient Preparation

The patient should not take aspirin, indomethacin, or anti-inflammatory medications, if possible, for at least 48 hours prior to collection of specimen.

Specimen Collection

Collect 3mL serum or EDTA plasma and separate as soon as possible. Freeze serum or plasma immediately after separation. Minimum specimen size is 1mL.

Special Specimens

For special fluids, such as CSF, vitreous fluid, peritoneal fluid, synovial fluid, contact ISI for requirements and special handling instructions.

Shipping Instructions

Ship specimens frozen in dry ice.

References
1. Redfern JS, Feldman M. Role of endogenous prostaglandins in preventing gastrointestinal ulceration: induction of ulcers by antibodies to prostaglandins. Gastroenterology.1989;Feb;96(2 Pt 2 Suppl):596-605.
2. Dunn MJ, Zambraski EJ. Renal effects of drugs that inhibit prostaglandin synthesis. Kidney Int. 1980;Nov;18(5):609-22.

CPT Code:
Prostaglandin E1 84150

PROSTAGLANDIN E2 (PG E2)

Reference Interval

250–400 pg/mL

Procedure

PG E2 is measured by radioimmunoassay/EIA/ELISA following extraction of specimens.

Patient Preparation

The patient should not take aspirin, indomethacin, or anti-inflammatory medications, if possible, for at least 48 hours prior to collection of specimen.

Specimen Collection

Collect 3mL serum or EDTA plasma and separate as soon as possible. Freeze serum or plasma immediately after separation. Minimum specimen size is 1mL.

Special Specimens

For special fluids, such as CSF, vitreous fluid, peritoneal fluid, synovial fluid, contact ISI for requirements and special handling instructions.

Shipping Instructions

Ship specimens frozen in dry ice.

References
1. Redfern JS, Feldman M. Role of endogenous prostaglandins in preventing gastrointestinal ulceration: induction of ulcers by antibodies to prostaglandins. Gastroenterology.1989;Feb;96(2 Pt 2 Suppl):596-605.
2. Balasch J, Arroyo V, Carmona F, et al. Severe ovarian hyperstimulation syndrome: role of peripheral vasodilation. Fertil Steril. 1991;Dec;56(6):1077-83.

CPT Code:
Prostaglandin E2 84150

PROSTAGLANDIN F2–α (PG F2–α)

Reference Interval

80–240 pg/mL

Procedure

PG F2-α is measured by radioimmunoassay/EIA/ELISA following extraction of specimens.

Patient Preparation

The patient should not take aspirin, indomethacin, or anti-inflammatory medications, if possible, for at least 48 hours prior to collection of specimen.

Specimen Collection

Collect 3 mL serum or EDTA plasma and separate as soon as possible. Freeze serum or plasma immediately after separation. Minimum specimen size is 1 mL.

Special Specimens

For special fluids, such as CSF, vitreous fluid, peritoneal fluid, synovial fluid, contact ISI for requirements and special handling instructions.

Shipping Instructions

Ship specimens frozen in dry ice.

References
1. Redfern JS, Feldman M. Role of endogenous prostaglandins in preventing gastrointestinal ulceration: induction of ulcers by antibodies to prostaglandins. Gastroenterology.1989;Feb;96(2 Pt 2 Suppl):596-605.
2. Bennegard B, Hahlin M, Hamberger L. Luteotropic effects of prostaglandins I2 and D2 on isolated human corpora luteum. Fertil Steril.1990;Sep;54(3):459-64.

CPT Code:
Prostaglandin F2-α 84150

SECRETIN

Reference Interval

12–75 pg/mL

Procedure

Secretin is measured by direct radioimmunoassay.

Patient Preparation

The patient should fast for 10 to 12 hours prior to collection of specimen. Antacid medications and medications that affect intestinal motility should be discontinued, if possible, for at least 48 hours prior to collection of specimen.

Specimen Collection

Collect 10mL blood directly into ISI's G.I. Preservative tube and separate as soon as possible. Freeze plasma immediately after separation. Special G.I. Preservative tubes are available from ISI. Minimum specimen size is 1mL.

Important Precaution

Secretin specimens must be collected using ISI's G.I. Preservative tube. No other methods of collection are acceptable.

Special Specimens

For special fluids, such as CSF, vitreous fluid, peritoneal fluid, synovial fluid, contact ISI for requirements and special handling instructions.

Shipping Instructions

Ship specimens frozen in dry ice.

References
1. Christ A, Werth B, Hildebrand P. Human secretin: biologic effects and plasma kinetics in humans. Gastroenterology.1988;Feb;94(2):311-6.
2. Yanaihara N, Sakagami M, Sato H, et al. Immunological aspects of secretin, substance P and VIP. 1977;Apr;72(4 Pt. 2):803-10.
3. Noda T, Ishikawa O, Eguchi H, et al. The diagnosis of pancreatic endocrine tumors.Gastroenterology.2004;62(5):907-10.
4. Hirst BH. Secretin and the exposition of hormonal control. J Physiol. 2004;15 Oct;560(Pt 2):339.
5. Chey WY, Chang TM. Secretin, 100 years later. J Gastroenterol.2003;38(11):1025-35.
6. Chey WY, Chang TM. Neural control of the release and action of secretin. J Physiol Pharmacol.2003;Dec;54(Suppl 4):105-12.
7. Konturek PC, Konturek SJ. The history of gastrointestinal hormones and the Polish contribution to elucidation of their biology and relation to nervous system. J Physiol Pharmacol.2003;54(Suppl 3):83-98.

CPT Code:
Unspecified Quantitative Immunoassay 83519

SEROTONIN (5-HT), SERUM

Reference Interval

Female:	80–450 ng/mL
Male:	40–400 ng/mL

Procedure

Serotonin is measured by direct radioimmunoassay.

Patient Preparation

The patient should fast for 10 to 12 hours prior to collection of specimen. Because of the diurnal variation of serotonin secretion, morning specimens are preferred.

Specimen Collection

Collect 5mL serum. Separate and freeze serum immediately after separation. Minimum specimen size is 1mL.

Important Precaution

For serotonin measurements, avoid hemolysis. Do not use a tourniquet. Handle specimens gently. Hemolysis results in spuriously high results.

Special Specimens

For special fluids, such as CSF, vitreous fluid, peritoneal fluid, synovial fluid, contact ISI for requirements and special handling instructions.

Shipping Instructions

Ship specimens frozen in dry ice.

References
1. Chauveau J, Fert V, Morel AM, et al. Rapid and specific enzyme immunoassay of serotonin. Clin Chem. 1991;37:1178-84.
2. Kellum JM Jr, Jaffe BM. Validation and application of a radioimmunoassay for serotonin. Gastroenterology.1976;Apr;70(4):516-22.
3. Donaldson D. Carcinoid tumours--the carcinoid syndrome and serotonin (5-HT): a brief review. J R Soc Health. 2000;Jun;120(2):78-9.

CPT Code:
Serotonin 84260

SOMATOSTATIN (SOMATOTROPIN RELEASE–INHIBITING FACTOR [SRIF])

Reference Interval

Up to 25 pg/mL

Procedure

Somatostatin is measured by direct radioimmunoassay.

Patient Preparation

The patient should fast for 10 to 12 hours prior to collection of specimen. The patient should not take any medications that affect insulin secretion or intestinal motility, if possible, for at least 48 hours prior to collection of specimen.

Specimen Collection

Collect 10mL blood directly into ISI's G.I. Preservative tube and separate as soon as possible. Freeze plasma immediately after separation. Special G.I. Preservative tubes are available from ISI. Minimum specimen size is 1mL.

Important Precaution

Somatostatin specimens must be collected using ISI's G.I. Preservative tube. No other methods of collection are acceptable.

Special Specimens

For special fluids, such as CSF, vitreous fluid, peritoneal fluid, synovial fluid, contact ISI for requirements and special handling instructions.

Shipping Instructions

Ship specimens frozen in dry ice.

References
1. Vinik AI, Gaginella TS, O'Dorisio TM, et al. The distribution and characterization of somatostatin-like immunoreactivity (SRIF- LI) in isolated cells, submucosa and muscle of the rat stomach and intestine. Endocrinology.1981;Dec;109(6):1921-6.
2. Hansen BC, Vinik A, Jen KL, et al. Fluctuations in basal levels and effects of altered nutrition on plasma somatostatin. Am J Physiol.1982;Sep;243(3):R289-95.
3. Lamberts SW. The role of somatostatin in the regulation of anterior pituitary hormone secretion and the use of its analogs in the treatment of human pituitary tumors. Endocr Rev. 1988; Nov;9(4):417-36.
4. Shoelson SE, Polonsky KS, Nakabayashi T. Circulating forms of somatostatinlike immunoreactivity in human plasma. Am J Physiol.1986;Apr;250(4 Pt 1):E428-34.
5. Low MJ. Clinical endocrinology and metabolism. The somatostatin neuroendocrine system: physiology and clinical relevance in gastrointestinal and pancreatic disorders. Best Pract Res Clin Endocrinol Metab.2004; 18(4):607-22.

CPT Code:
Somatostatin 84307

SUBSTANCE P

Reference Interval

40–270 pg/mL

Procedure

Substance P is measured by direct radioimmunoassay.

Patient Preparation

The patient should fast 10 to 12 hours prior to collection of specimen. Antacid medications and medications that affect intestinal motility should be discontinued, if possible, for at least 48 hours prior to collection of specimen.

Specimen Collection

Collect 10mL blood directly into ISI's Z-tube™ Preservative and separate as soon as possible. Freeze plasma immediately after separation. Special Z-tube™ Preservatives are available from ISI. Minimum specimen size is 1mL.

Important Precaution

Substance P plasma specimens must be collected using ISI's Z-tube™ Preservative. No other methods of collection are acceptable

Special Specimens

*Frozen Z-tube™ plasma is the only acceptable sample type for this assay.

Shipping Instructions

Ship specimens frozen in dry ice.

References
1. Aronin N, Leeman SE, Clements RS Jr. Diminished flare response in neuropathic diabetic patients: comparison of effects of substance P, histamine and capsaicin. Diabetes.1987;Oct;36(10):1139-43.
2. Aronin N, Coslovsky R, Chase K. Hypothyroidism increases substance P concentrations in the heterotropic anterior pituitary. Endocrinology.1988;Jun;122(6):2911-4.
3. Vinik AI, Gonin J, England BG, et al. Plasma substance-P in neuroendocrine tumors and idiopathic flushing: the value of pentagastrin stimulation tests and the effects of somatostatin analog.J Clin Endocrinol Metab. 1990;70(6):1702-9.

CPT Code:
Unspecified Quantitative Immunoassay 83519

THROMBOXANE B$_2$ (TxB$_2$)

Reference Interval

180–420 pg/mL

Procedure

Thromboxane B$_2$ is measured by radioimmunoassay following extraction of specimens.

Patient Preparation

The patient should not take aspirin, indomethacin, or anti-inflammatory medications for at least 48 hours prior to collection of specimen. Fasting patients may have elevated levels of thromboxane B$_2$.

Specimen Collection

Collect 3mL EDTA plasma and separate as soon as possible. Freeze plasma immediately after separation. Minimum specimen size is 1mL.

Special Specimens

For special fluids, such as CSF, vitreous fluid, peritoneal fluid, synovial fluid, contact ISI for requirements and special handling instructions.

Shipping Instructions

Ship specimens frozen in dry ice.

References
1. Gonzalez-Revalderia J, Sabater J, et al. Usefulness of thromboxane B$_2$ in diagnosis of renal transplant rejection. Clin Chem. 1991;Dec;37(12):2157.
2. Willerson JT, Eidt JF, McNatt J, et al. Role of thromboxane and serotonin as mediators in the development of spontaneous alterations in coronary blood flow and neointimal proliferation in canine models with chronic coronary artery stenoses and endothelial injury. J Am Coll Cardiol.1991;May;17(6 Suppl B):101B-10B.

CPT Code:
Unspecified Quantitative Immunoassay 83519

THROMBOXANE B$_2$ (TxB$_2$), URINE

Reference Interval

50–160 ng/24 hours

Procedure

Thromboxane B$_2$ is measured by radioimmunoassay following extraction of specimens.

Patient Preparation

The patient should not take aspirin, indomethacin, or anti-inflammatory medications for at least 48 hours prior to collection of specimen. Fasting patients may have elevated levels of Thromboxane B$_2$.

Specimen Collection

Submit 5mL of a 24-hour urine collection. No special preservatives are required. Minimum specimen size is 1mL. Provide total volume per 24 hours, if possible; however, random urine samples are acceptable.

Shipping Instructions

Ship specimens frozen in dry ice.

References
1. Gonzalez-Revalderia J, Sabater J, Villafruela JJ, et al. Usefulness of thromboxane B$_2$ in diagnosis of renal transplant rejection. Clin Chem.1991;Dec;37(12):2157.
2. Willerson JT, Eidt JF, McNatt J, et al. Role of thromboxane and serotonin as mediators in the development of spontaneous alterations in coronary blood flow and neointimal proliferation in canine models with chronic coronary artery stenoses and endothelial injury.J Am Coll Cardiol.1991;May;17(6 Suppl B):101B-10B.

CPT Code:
Unspecified Quantitative Immunoassay 83519

THYROTROPIN RELEASING HORMONE (TRH)

Reference Interval

Up to 40 pg/mL

Procedure

TRH is measured by direct radioimmunoassay.

Patient Preparation

The patient should not take any thyroid medication, if possible, for at least 48 hours prior to collection of specimen.

Specimen Collection

Collect 10mL blood directly into ISI's TRH Preservative tube and separate as soon as possible. Freeze plasma immediately after separation. Special TRH Preservative tubes are available from ISI. Minimum specimen size is 1mL.

Important Precaution

TRH plasma specimens must be collected using ISI's TRH Preservative tube. No other methods of collection are acceptable

Special Specimens

*Frozen TRH plasma is the only acceptable sample type for this assay.

Shipping Instructions

Ship specimens frozen in dry ice.

References
1. Kaplan MM, Taft JA, Reichlin S, et al. Sustained rises in serum thyrotropin, thyroxine, and triiodothyronine during long term, continuous thyrotropin-releasing hormone treatment in patients with amyotrophic lateral sclerosis. J Clin Endocrinol Metab.1986;Oct;63(4):808-14.
2. Shambaugh GE III, Wilber JF, Montoya E, et al. Thyrotropin-releasing hormone (TRH): measurement in human spinal fluid. J Clin Endocrinol Metab.1975;Jul;41(1):131-4.

CPT Code:
Unspecified Quantitative Immunoassay 83519

THYROTROPIN RELEASING HORMONE (TRH), URINE

Reference Interval

2 – 40 ng/24 hours.

Procedure

TRH is measured by direct radioimmunoassay.

Patient Preparation

The patient should not take any thyroid medication, if possible, for at least 48 hours prior to collection of specimen.

Specimen Collection

Submit 5mL of a well mixed 24-hour urine collection. No special preservatives are required. Minimum specimen size is 1mL. Provide total volume per 24 hours, if possible; however, random urine samples are acceptable.

Shipping Instructions

Ship specimens frozen in dry ice.

References
1. Kaplan MM, Taft JA, Reichlin S, et al. Sustained rises in serum thyrotropin, thyroxine, and triiodothyronine during long term, continuous thyrotropin-releasing hormone treatment in patients with amyotrophic lateral sclerosis. J Clin Endocrinol Metab.1986;Oct;63(4):808-14.
2. Shambaugh GE III, Wilber JF, Montoya E, et al. Thyrotropin-releasing hormone (TRH): measurement in human spinal fluid. J Clin Endocrinol Metab.1975;Jul;41(1):131-4.

CPT Code:
Unspecified Quantitative Immunoassay 83519

VASOACTIVE INTESTINAL POLYPEPTIDE (VIP)

Reference Interval

Up to 36 pg/mL

Procedure

VIP is measured by direct radioimmunoassay.

Patient Preparation

The patient should fast for 10 to 12 hours prior to collection of specimen. Antacid medications and medications that affect intestinal motility should be discontinued, if possible, for at least 48 hours prior to collection of specimen.

Specimen Collection

Collect 10mL blood directly into ISI's G.I. Preservative tube and separate as soon as possible. Freeze plasma immediately after separation. Special G.I. Preservative tubes are available from ISI. Minimum specimen size is 1mL.

Important Precaution

VIP specimens must be collected using ISI's G.I. Preservative tube. No other methods of collection are acceptable.

Special Specimens

For special fluids, such as CSF, vitreous, peritoneal fluid, synovial fluid, contact ISI for requirements and special handling instructions.

Shipping Instructions

Ship specimens frozen in dry ice.

References
1. O'Dorisio MS, Wood CL, O'Dorisio TM. Vasoactive intestinal peptide and neuropeptide modulation of the immune response. J Immunol.1985;Aug;135(2 Suppl):792S-6S.
2. Ollerenshaw S, Jarvis D, Woolcock A, et al. Absence of immunoreactive vasoactive intestinal polypeptide in tissue from the lungs of patients with asthma. N Engl J Med.1989;11 May;320(19):1244-8.
3. Palsson OS, Morteau O, Bozymski EM, et al. Elevated vasoactive intestinal peptide concentrations in patients with irritable bowel syndrome. Dig Dis Sci. 2004;49(7-8):1236-43.
4. Gomariz RP, Martinez C, Abad C, et al. Immunology of VIP: a review and therapeutical perspectives. Curr Pharm Des.2001;7(2):89-111.
5. Gozes I, Furman S. Clinical endocrinology and metabolism. Potential clinical applications of vasoactive intestinal peptide: a selected update. Best Pract Res Clin Endocrinol Metab. 2001; 18(4):623-40.
6. Kodali S, Ding W, Huang J, et al. Vasoactive intestinal peptide modulates langerhans cell immune function. J Immunol.2004;173(10):6082-88.

CPT Code:
Vasoactive Intestinal Polypeptide 84586

VASOACTIVE INTESTINAL POLYPEPTIDE (VIP), URINE

Reference Interval

Up to 70 ng/24 hours.

Procedure

VIP is measured by direct radioimmunoassay.

Patient Preparation

Antacid medications and medications that affect intestinal motility should be discontinued, if possible, for at least 48 hours prior to collection of specimen.

Specimen Collection

Submit 5mL of a well mixed 24-hour urine collection. No special preservatives are required. Minimum specimen size is 1mL. Provide total volume per 24 hours, if possible; however, random urine samples are acceptable.

Shipping Instructions

Ship specimens frozen in dry ice.

References

1. O'Dorisio MS, Wood CL, O'Dorisio TM. Vasoactive intestinal peptide and neuropeptide modulation of the immune response. J Immunol. 1985;Aug;135(2 Suppl):792S-6S.
2. Ollerenshaw S, Jarvis D, Woolcock A, et al. Absence of immunoreactive vasoactive intestinal polypeptide in tissue from the lungs of patients with asthma. N Engl J Med.1989; 11 May;320(19):1244-8.
3. Palsson OS, Morteau O, Bozymski EM, et al. Elevated vasoactive intestinal peptide concentrations in patients with irritable bowel syndrome. Dig Dis Sci. 2004;49(7-8):1236-43.
4. Gomariz RP, Martinez C, Abad C, et al. Immunology of VIP: a review and therapeutical perspectives. Curr Pharm Des. 2001; 7(2):89-111.
5. Gozes I, Furman S. Clinical endocrinology and metabolism. Potential clinical applications of vasoactive intestinal peptide: a
6. Kodali S, Ding W, Huang J, et al. Vasoactive intestinal peptide modulates langerhans cell immune function. J Immunol. 2004;173(10):6082-88.

CPT Code:
Vasoactive Intestinal Polypeptide 84586

TESTS AVAILABLE BY REQUEST ONLY*

- Brain Natiuretic Peptide (BNP)
- C-Reactive Peptide
- Calcitonin
- Carboxy-Methyl Lysine
- Exendin
- Fibrinogen
- Galanin
- Homocysteine
- Free Insulin
- Insulin antibodies
- Nuclear Factor Kappa Beta (NFK-b)
- Oxytocin
- Proinsulin
- Prostaglandins: PG F2-Alpha; 6-Keto PG F1-Alpha & Dihydroketo PG E2

*Contact ISI for availability of these or any other tests not currently listed in this handbook or on the web.

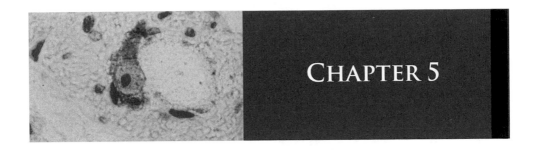

CHAPTER 5

PROFILES, INCLUDING CPT CODES

BASIC NETS/CARCINOID FOLLOW-UP PROFILE

Measure every 3 months or immediately following a therapeutic intervention.

BLOOD
- 5HIAA (Plasma)
- CgA
- Neurokinin A (NKA)
- Pancreastatin
- Substance P

If on Sandostatin LAR® for at least three months, consider measuring (immediately prior to the LAR® injection):
- Octreotide

If on Somatuline® Depot for four months or longer, consider measuring (immediately prior to the next injection):
- Lanreotide

For increase in tumor growth or rise in biomarkers, consider other amines, peptides, and markers found to be elevated in the screening evaluation profile.

URINE
Measure every 3–6 months or immediately following a therapeutic intervention.
- 5-HIAA (or 5-HTP if 5-HIAA is negative and 5-HTP is positive at initial screening)

Patient Preparation

Patient should fast overnight prior to collection of blood specimens. Because of the diurnal variation of serotonin secretion, morning specimens are preferred. For the pancreastatin assay, patients should be advised to discontinue medications that affect insulin levels, if possible, for 48 hours prior to collection. Patients should not partake of the following foods for 48 hours prior to collection of <u>urine</u> for measurement of 5-HIAA and 5-HTP. (*However, if the 5-HIAA plasma assay is utilized, fasting from these foods is only required for 8 hours.*)
- Red wine
- Cheese
- Hot dogs
- Chocolates
- Vanilla-containing foods (e.g., ice cream)
- Custard
- Pineapple, kiwi, bananas, cassava
- Avocado
- Tomato
- Walnuts

Specimen Requirements

BLOOD & URINE
See individual test listings (Chapter 4, Assays) for applicable patient preparation, specimen requirements and shipping instructions. For tests not listed, contact your contracted laboratory for applicable requirements.

References
1. Oberg K, Kvols L, Caplin M, et al. Consensus report of the use of somatostatin analogs for the management of neuroendocrine tumors of the gastroenteropancreatic system. Ann Oncol. 2004; Jun;15(6):966-73.
2. Please refer to www.nccn.org, The National Comprehensive Cancer Network clinical practice guidelines in oncology.

CPT Codes: Blood
5-HIAA (Plasma) 82542
Chromogranin A 86316
Serotonin 84260
Pancreastatin 83519
Octreotide 80299
Neurokinin A 83519
Substance P 83519

CPT Codes: Urine
5-HIAA Random Urine 83497, 82570
5-HIAA 24-Hour Urine 83497
5-HTP 86316

BRONCHOSPASM PROFILE

This profile is useful for ruling out a neuroendocrine tumor cause of bronchospasm.

BLOOD
- 5-HIAA
- Prostaglandin D2
- Histamine
- Serotonin
- Substance P
- VIP
- CgA
- Pancreastatin
- Serum protein immunoelectrophoresis, IgE

URINE
- 5-HIAA (if blood levels are not used)
- 5-HTP
- VMA
- Tryptase

Patient Preparation

The patient should fast for 10 to 12 hours prior to collection of specimen. Alkali antacid medications should be discontinued, if possible, for at least 24 hours prior to collection. PPIs and H2 blockers should be discontinued for 72 hours or more prior to collection and patients monitored closely. For 48 hours prior to sample collection, patients should not be treated with the following medications, if possible:
- Insulin or oral medications that influence insulin production or secretion
- Aspirin, indomethacin, or anti-inflammatory medications
- Antacids or medications affecting intestinal motility

Patients should not partake of the following foods for 48 hours prior to collection of urine for measurement of 5-HIAA and 5-HTP. *(However, if the 5-HIAA plasma assay is utilized, fasting from these foods is only required for 8 hours.)*
- Red wine
- Cheese
- Hot dogs
- Chocolates
- Vanilla-containing foods (e.g., ice cream)
- Custard
- Pineapple, kiwi, bananas, or cassava
- Avocado
- Tomato
- Walnuts

Specimen Requirements

BLOOD & URINE
See individual test listings (Chapter 4, Assays) for applicable patient preparation, specimen requirements and shipping instructions. For tests not listed, contact your contracted laboratory for applicable requirements.

Further Diagnosis

Refer patient for allergy testing.

Reference
1. Chughtai TS, Morin JE, Sheiner NM, et al. Bronchial Carcinoid—20 years experience defines a selective surgical approach. Surgery.1997;Oct;122(4):801-8.

CPT Codes: Blood
5-HIAA (Plasma) 82542
Prostaglandin D_2 84150
Histamine 83088
Serotonin 84260
Substance P 83159
VIP 84686
Chromogranin A 86316
Pancreastatin 83519
Serum Protein Immunoelectrophoresis IgE 86003

CPT Codes: Urine
5-HIAA 24-Hour Urine 83497
5-HTP 86316
Vanillyl mandelic acid (VMA) 84585

DIARRHEA SYNDROME TESTS

BLOOD
- 5-HIAA
- VIP
- Gastrin
- Gastrin-releasing peptide
- Calcitonin (MCT)
- PG D2
- Histamine
- CgA
- Pancreastatin
- Pancreatic polypeptide (PP)
- PTH and PTHrp if hypercalcemic
- CGRP and substance P if flushing
- Plasma 5-HIAA
- Plasma Free metanephrines (if hypertensive)

URINE
- 5-HIAA (if blood levels are not used)
- 5-HTP
- VMA and catecholamines if hypertensive

STOOL

Measurement of stool electrolytes and osmolarity should be done early in the diagnostic evaluation. The presence of an osmolar gap suggests factitious diarrhea. A 72-hour supervised fast with intravenous fluid administration may also help determine if the diarrhea is secretory or infectious.

Patient Preparation

Patient should fast for 10 to 12 hours prior to collection of blood specimen. Antacid medications, anti-histamine medications, aspirin, indomethacin, anti-inflammatory medications, and medications affecting motility or pancreatic function should be discontinued, if possible, for at least 48 hours prior to collection. Patients should not partake of the following foods for 48 hours prior to collection of urine for measurement of 5-HIAA and 5-HT. *(However, if the 5-HIAA plasma assay is utilized, fasting from these foods is only required for 8 hours.)*
- Red wine
- Cheese
- Hot dogs
- Chocolates
- Vanilla-containing foods (e.g., ice cream)
- Custard
- Pineapple, kiwi, bananas, cassava
- Avocado
- Tomato
- Walnuts

Specimen Requirements

BLOOD & URINE
See individual test listings (Chapter 4, Assays) for applicable patient preparation, specimen requirements and shipping instructions. For tests not listed, contact your contracted laboratory for applicable requirements.

References
1. Vinik AI, Tsai ST, Moattari AR, et al. Somatostatin analog (SMS 201-995) in the management of gastroenteropancreatic tumors and diarrhea syndromes. Am J Med. 1986; 81(6B):23-40.
2. Verner JV, Morrison AB. Islet cell tumor and a syndrome of refractory watery diarrhea and hypokalemia. Am J Med. 1958;25(3):374-80.
3. Murray JS, Paton RR, Pope CE. Pancreatic tumor associated with flushing and diarrhea. Report of a case. N Engl J Med. 1961;264:436-9.
4. Arnold R, Lankisch PG. Somatostatin and the gastrointestinal tract. Clin Gastroenterol. 1980; 9(3):733-53.
5. Stockmann F, Richter G, Lembeke B, Conlon JM, Creutzfeldt W. Long-term treatment of patients with endocrine gastrointestinal tumors with the somatostatin analog SMS 201-995. Scand J Gastroenterol. 1986; 21:230.
6. Hengl G, Prager J, Pointner H. The influence of somatostatin on the absorption of triglycerides in partially gastrectomized subjects. Acta Hepatogastroenterol (Stuttg). 1979; Oct;26(5):392-5.
7. Vinik A, Moattari AR. Use of somatostatin analog in management of carcinoid syndrome. Dig Dis Sci. 1989; 34(3 Suppl):14S-27S.

CPT Codes: Blood
5-HIAA (Plasma) 82542
Vasoactive Intestinal Polypeptide (VIP) 84686
Gastrin 82938-82941
Bombesin 83519
Calcitonin 82308
Prostaglandin D$_2$ 84150
Histamine 83088
Chromogranin A 86316
Pancreastatin 83519
Pancreatic Polypeptide 83519
PTH 83519
PTHRP 83519
CGRP: Unlisted Chemistry Procedure 84999 or Unspecified Immunoassay 83520
Substance P 83519

CPT Codes: Urine
5-HIAA 83497
5-HTP 86701
Vanillyl mandelic acid (VMA) 84585
Catecholamines 82384

DUMPING SYNDROME

BASAL/FASTING TESTS
Following an overnight fast, patients should have blood drawn for the following tests:
- Pancreatic polypeptide (PP)
- Glucagon
- GLP-1, Total
- Insulin
- Motilin
- GIP

FECAL MEASUREMENTS
- Fecal Elastase (EL-1)
- Fecal fat measurement
- Fecal chymotrypsin measurement

Patient Preparation

Patients should fast for 10 to 12 hours prior to collection of specimens. Patients should discontinue medications that affect insulin production or secretion, antacid medications, or medications affecting intestinal motility, if possible, for 48 hours prior to collection.

Specimen Collection

BLOOD & URINE
See individual test listings (Chapter 4, Assays) for applicable patient preparation, specimen requirements and shipping instructions. For tests not listed, contact your local hospital or contracted laboratory for applicable requirements.

STOOL
Collect 100 mg of formed stool and store at –20°C. Stool specimens are stable for 7 days at refrigerated temperatures. Minimum specimen size is 20 mg of formed stool. Note on request slip if sample has watery diarrhea consistency, as concentration levels of Fecal Elastase (EL-1) may be decreased due to dilution factor.

CPT Codes:
GLP-1, Total 83519
Insulin 83525 • Proinsulin 84206 • Proinsulin Serum 84206
Motilin 83519
Amylase 82150
Lipase 83690
Trypsin 84488
Fecal Fat • Quantitative 82710 • Qualitative 82705
Fecal Chymotrypsin 84311
Fecal Elastase 1 82656
GIP 83519

References
1. Harris AG, O'Dorisio TM, Woltering EA, et al. Consensus statement: octreotide dose titration in secretory diarrhea. Diarrhea Management Consensus Development Panel. Dig Dis Sci. 1995;Jul;40(7):1464-73.
2. Mozell EJ, Woltering EA, O'Dorisio TM. Non-endocrine applications of somatostatin and octreotide acetate: facts and flights of fancy. Dis Mon. 1991;Dec;37(12):749-848.
3. Richards WO, Geer R, O'Dorisio TM, et al. Octreotide acetate induces fasting small bowel motility in patients with dumping syndrome. J Surg Res. 1990; Dec;49(6):483-7.
4. Geer RJ, Richards WO, O'Dorisio TM, et al. Efficacy of octreotide acetate in treatment of severe postgastrectomy dumping syndrome. Ann Surg. 1990;Dec;212(6):678-87.
5. Woltering EA, O'Dorisio TM, Williams ST, et al. Treatment of nonendocrine gastrointestinal disorders with octreotide acetate. Metabolism. 1990; Sep;39(9 Suppl 2):176-9.

Flushing Syndrome Tests

Tests to Identify Causes of Flushing in Different Clinical Syndromes

Clinical Condition	Tests
Carcinoid	5-HIAA (plasma or urine), 5-HTP, substance P, CGRP, CgA
MCT	Calcitonin, calcium infusion, RET protooncogene
Pheochromocytoma	VMA, epinephrine, norepinephrine, dopamine, glucagon stimulation test, T2-weighted MRI, OctreoScan®,[131]I-MIBG
Diabetic autonomic neuropathy	Heart rate variability, 2-hour postprandial glucose
Menopause	FSH
Epilepsy	Electroencephalogram
Panic syndrome	Pentagastrin-stimulated ACTH
Mastocytosis	Histamine (plasma), VIP, tryptase (urine)
Hypomastia, mitral prolapse	Echocardiography

BLOOD
- 5-HIAA (Plasma)
- CgA
- Pancreastatin
- Substance P
- VIP
- Gastrin
- Neurotensin
- Serotonin
- CGRP
- Calcitonin
- FSH
- Histamine
- Plasma Free metanephrines (if hypertensive)

URINE
For all 24-hour urine collections, measure creatinine.
- 5-HIAA *(if blood levels are not used)*
- 5-HTP
- VMA if hypertensive
- Tryptase

CONSIDER
- Plasma catecholamines if hypertensive
- Dopamine
- Epinephrine
- Norepinephrine
- PTH and PTHRP if hypercalcemic
- MEN screen (gastrin, prolactin, pancreatic polypeptide, and ionized Ca++)
- MEN-1 gene and RET protooncogene
- Calcitonin, gastrin, and ACTH for degree of tumor aggression
- CA 19-1
- BNP, otherwise known as atrial natriuretic factor, if echocardiogram abnormal

ADDITIONAL TESTING IN PATIENTS WITH UNUSUAL CLINICAL SYNDROMES
- GH-RH
- Bombesin
- Ghrelin, Total
- IGF-1, IGF-2
- Corticotropin-releasing factor (CRF)

TISSUE STAINS (tumor must be proven histologically before these stains are done)
- Ki-67
- CgA
- Synaptophysin

CONSIDER
- Factor VIII, CD 31, AE1/AE3
- Somatostatin receptor subtypes other than type 2
- NSE
- Somatostatin receptor type 2

Patient Preparation

Patient should fast overnight prior to collection of blood specimens. Antacid medications and medications affecting motility should be discontinued, if possible for at least 48 hours prior to collection of specimens. Patients should not partake of the following foods for 48 hours prior to collection of urine for measurement of 5-HIAA and 5-HTP measurements. *(However, if the 5-HIAA plasma assay is utilized, fasting from these foods is only required for 8 hours.)*
- Red wine
- Cheese
- Hot dogs
- Chocolates
- Vanilla-containing foods (e.g., ice cream)
- Custard
- Pineapple, kiwi, bananas, cassava
- Avocado
- Tomato
- Walnuts

Specimen Requirements

BLOOD & URINE
See individual test listings (Chapter 4, Assays) for applicable patient preparation, specimen requirements and shipping instructions. For tests not listed, contact your contracted laboratory for applicable requirements.

TISSUE
Consult specialist for tissue staining requirements.

References

1. Vinik AI, Tsai ST, Moattari AR, et al. Somatostatin analog (SMS 201-995) in the management of gastroenteropancreatic tumors and diarrhea syndromes. Am J Med. 1988;81(6B):23-40.
2. Verner JV, Morrison AB. Islet cell tumor and a syndrome of refractory watery diarrhea and hypokalemia. Am J Med. 1958;25(3):374-80.
3. Murray JS, Paton RR, Pope CE. Pancreatic tumor associated with flushing and diarrhea. Report of a case. N Engl J Med. 1961;264:436-9.
4. Arnold R, Lankisch PG. Somatostatin and the gastrointestinal tract. Clin Gastroenterol. 1980;9(3):733-53.
5. Stockmann F, Richter G, Lembeke B, et al. Long-term treatment of patients with endocrine gastrointestinal tumors with the somatostatin analog SMS 201-995. Scand J Gastroenterol. 1986;2:230.
6. Hengl G, Prager J, Pointner H. The influence of somatostatin on the absorption of triglycerides in partially gastrectomized subjects. Acta Hepatogastroenterol (Stuttg). 1979;26(5):392-5.
7. Vinik A, Moattari AR. Use of somatostatin analog in management of carcinoid syndrome. Dig Dis Sci. 1989;34(3 Suppl):14S-27S.

CPT Codes:

Urine
- 5-HIAA 24-Hour Urine 83497
- 5-HTP 86316
- VMA 84585
- Tryptase 83520

5-HIAA (Plasma) 82542

Calcitonin 82308

Epinephrine 82383

Norepinephrine 82491

FSH 83001

ACTH 82024

Histamine 83088

Substance P 83519

Gastrin 82938-82941

VIP 84686

Neurotensin 83519

Chromogranin A 86316

Calcium 82310

Catecholamines 82384

PTH 83519

PTH RP 83519

BNP 83880

Growth Hormone–Releasing Hormone 83519

Bombesin 83519

IGF-1 84305

IGF-2 83520

Ghrelin 83519

CRF 83519

Enolase 86316

MEN Type 1 Screen
- Gastrin 82938–82941
- Prolactin 84146
- Pancreatic Polypeptide 83519
- Iolonized Calcium 82330

Glucagon 82943
- Tolerance Panel 80422–80424
- Tolerance Test 82946

Insulin 83525
- Proinsulin 84206
- Proinsulin Serum 84206

GASTRINOMA (ZOLLINGER-ELLISON) SCREEN

BASAL/FASTING TESTS
- Fasting gastrin concentration
- Chromogranin A (CgA)
- Pancreastatin
- Gastric pH

CONSIDER
- Pancreatic polypeptide (PP) for pancreatic location and suspected MEN-1
- MEN-1 screen
- ACTH if rapid tumor growth, history of hypertension, diabetes, bruising, or Cushing's syndrome.
- OctreoScan and CT or MRI

Patient Preparation

Patient should fast for 10 to 12 hours prior to collection of specimen. Alkali antacid medications should be discontinued, if possible, for at least 24 hours prior to collection. PPIs and H2 blockers should be discontinued for 72 hours prior to collection and patients monitored closely.

Specimen Collection

BLOOD & URINE
See individual test listings (Chapter 4, Assays) for applicable patient preparation, specimen requirements and shipping instructions. For tests not listed, contact your contracted laboratory for applicable requirements.

References
1. Trudeau WI, McGuigan JE. Effects of calcium on serum gastrin levels in the Zollinger-Ellison syndrome. N Engl J Med. 1969;Oct;281(16):862-6.
2. Mozell EJ, Woltering EA, O'Dorisio TM, et al. Effect of somatostatin analog on peptide release and tumor growth in the Zollinger-Ellison syndrome. Surg Gynecol Obstet 1990;Jun;170(6):476-84.
3. Mozell EJ, Cramer AJ, O'Dorisio TM, et al. Long-term efficacy of octreotide in the treatment of Zollinger-Ellison syndrome. Arch Surg. 1992;Sep;127(9):1019-24, discussion 1024-6.
4. Mignon, M. Diagnostic and therapeutic strategies in Zollinger-Ellison syndrome associated with multiple endocrine neoplasia type I (MEN-I): experience of the Zollinger-Ellison Syndrome Research Group: Bichat 1958-1999. Bull Acad Nat Med. 2003;187(7):1249-58.
5. Mozell EJ, Woltering EA, O'Dorisio TM, et al. Effect of somatostatin analog on peptide release and tumor growth in the Zollinger-Ellison syndrome. Surg Gynecol Obstet. 1990;Jun;170(6):476-84.
6. Owyang C, Vinik AI. Diabetic pseudo Zollinger-Ellison syndrome. Gastroenterol. 1982;82(5):1144.

CPT Codes:
Gastrin 82941
ACTH 82024
Pancreatic Polypeptide 83519
MEN Type 1 Screen • Gastrin 82938–82941 • Prolactin 84146 • Pancreatic Polypeptide 83519 • Ionized Calcium 82330

GENERIC FOLLOW-UP PROFILES
PANCREAS AND MEN TESTS

BLOOD
- Ca++ corrected for albumin concentrations
- Every 3 months, measure specific peptides found to be elevated on screening profile
- Check other components of MEN syndrome screen for MEN measurements (see previous page)

CONSIDER
Fasting insulin if hypoglycaemic
- Octreotide suppression test, a predictive test for responsiveness to somatostatin analog therapy
- Octreotide levels for patients on drug, if patient symptoms, tumor, and biochemical markers are not responding
- RET protooncogene and MEN-1 gene (MENIN) if not tested previously

Patient Preparation

Patient should fast for 10 to 12 hours prior to collection of specimen. Alkali antacid medications should be discontinued, if possible, for at least 24 hours prior to collection. PPIs and H2 blockers should be discontinued for 72 hours prior to collection and patients monitored closely.

Specimen Requirements:

BLOOD & URINE
See individual test listings (Chapter 4, Assays) for applicable patient preparation, specimen requirements and shipping instructions. For tests not listed, contact your local hospital or contracted laboratory for applicable requirements.

References
1. Mozell EJ, Woltering EA, O'Dorisio TM, et al. Effect of somatostatin analog on peptide release and tumor growth in the Zollinger-Ellison syndrome. Surg Gynecol Obstet. 1990;Jun;170(6):476-84.
2. Mozell EJ, Woltering EA, O'Dorisio TM, et al. Adult onset nesidioblastosis: response of glucose, insulin, and secondary peptides to therapy with Sandostatin. Am J Gastroenterol. 1990;Feb;85(2):181-8.
3. Please refer to www.endotext.org.

CPT Codes
Octreotide 80299
MEN Type 1 Screen • Gastrin 82938-82941 • Insulin 83525 • Intact pTH • Prolactin 84146 • Pancreatic Polypeptide 83519 • Ionized Calcium 82330

GENETIC STUDIES

Neuroendocrine Tumors

BLOOD
- MEN-1 (MENIN gene)
- RET protooncogene (MEN-2)

Type 1 Diabetes

BLOOD
- HLA
- DR3
- DR4
- A2

Risk Factors for Diabetic Complications

- Superoxide dismutase gene polymorphism
- Toll receptor polymorphism
- ApoE gene polymorphism
- Angiotensin receptor gene polymorphism
- Glut 4 abnormalities
- Hepatic nuclear transcription factor 1 and 4 (MODY)
- Aldose reductase gene polymorphism (Z2 allele)
- Cytochrome P450 polymorphism
- TNFα gene polymorphism
- 5' Lipoxygenase gene polymorphism
- Mitochondrial DNA mutations
- Glucokinase gene abnormalities
- Mitochondrial DNA

Patient Preparation

Consult specialist for patient preparation.

Specimen Requirements

Consult specialist for specimen requirements.

Shipping Instructions

Consult specialist for shipping instructions.

Reference
1. Please refer to www.endotext.org.

GI–Neuroendocrine Tests

BLOOD
- 5-HIAA (Plasma)
- Neurotensin
- Ghrelin
- PTH
- PTHrp
- Prolactin
- Glucagon
- Insulin (if history of hypoglycemia) IGF I and IGF II
- C-Peptide (if history of hypoglycemia)
- Somatostatin
- Calcitonin
- VIP
- Gastrin
- Catecholamines (dopamine, epinephrine and norepinephrine if hypertensive)
- Plasma Free metanephrines (if hypertensive)

Patient Preparation

Patient should be fasting 10 to 12 hours prior to collection of specimen. Antacid medication, Corticosteroid, ACTH, Thyroid, Estrogen or Gonadotropin medications and medications affecting motility, gastrointestinal or pancreatic function should be discontinued, if possible, for at least 48 hours prior to collection.

URINE
- VMA if hypertensive
- Catecholamines [dopamine, epinephrine, (metaepinephrine) norepinephrine (normetanephrine) if hypertensive]

Specimen Requirements

BLOOD & URINE
See individual test listings (Chapter 4, Assays) for applicable patient preparation, specimen requirements and shipping instructions. For tests not listed, contact your local hospital or contracted laboratory for applicable requirements.

References
1. Please refer to Aaron I. Vinik in www.endotext.org/guthormones/index.htm.

CPT Codes:
5-HIAA (Plasma) 82542
Neurotensin 83519
Ghrelin 83519
PTH 83519
PTH-Related Peptide 83519
Prolactin 84146
Glucagon 82943 • Tolerance Panel 80422–80424 • Tolerance Test 82946
Insulin 83525
IGF-1 84305
IGF-2 83520
C-Peptide
Somatostatin 84307
Calcitonin 82308
VIP 84686
Gastrin 82938–82941
Catecholamines 82384
Dopamine 82384
Epinephrine 82383
Norepinephrine 82491
Insulin 80422, 80432–80435 • Antibody 86337 • Blood 83525 • Free 83527
Plasma free metanephrines 83835

HYPOGLYCEMIA/INSULINOMA SCREENING TEST

Patient Preparation

Patients should be advised to discontinue medications that affect insulin levels, if possible, for 48 hours prior to collection. After an overnight fast, basal blood samples are collected to measure the following:

- Insulin
- Proinsulin
- C-peptide
- IGF-1 and IGF-2

Specimen Requirements

BLOOD
See individual test listings (Chapter 4, Assays) for applicable patient preparation, specimen requirements and shipping instructions. For tests not listed, contact your local hospital or contracted laboratory for applicable requirements.

Reference
1. Fajans SS, Vinik AI. Diagnosis and treatment of "insulinoma." In: Santen RJ, Manni A, eds. Diagnosis and Management of Endocrine-Related Tumors. Boston, MA: Martinus Nijhoff Publishers; 1984:235.

©2006 Inter Science Institute. This profile of assays for the hypoglycemia insulinoma screening has been copyrighted.

CPT Codes:
Insulin 83525
Proinsulin 84206
Proinsulin Serum 84206
C-Peptide 84681
IGF-1 84305
IGF-2 83520

LIPOPROTEIN PROFILE
(TOTAL CHOLESTEROL, HDL-C, LDL-C, PARTICLE SIZE, AND TRIGLYCERIDES)

Lipoprotein profile (either VAP™ or NMR method)
- Triglycerides
- Total cholesterol
- HDL-C
- LDL-C
- LDL-C particle size

Patient Preparation

Consult local laboratory for patient preparation.

Specimen Requirements

Consult local laboratory for specimen requirements.

Shipping Instructions

Consult local laboratory for shipping instructions.

Reference
 1. Please refer to www.endotext.org.

CPT Codes:
HDL-C 83718
LDL-C 83721
Particle Size 83704
Total Cholesterol 82465
Triglycerides 84478

MEN SYNDROME TYPE 1 AND 2 SCREEN

BLOOD
- 5-HIAA (Plasma)
- Pituitary (MEN-1)
    - Prolactin
    - Growth hormone if features of acromegaly
- Parathyroid (MEN-1 and -2)
    - PTH
    - PTHRP
    - Ionized Ca++ or Ca++ corrected for serum albumin
    - 24-Hour urine collection for Ca++ and PO
- Pancreas (MEN-1)
    - Pancreatic polypeptide (PP)
    - Gastrin
    - Insulin/C-peptide if patient hypoglycemic
    - CgA
- Thyroid C cells (MEN-2)
    - Calcitonin
    - CEA
- Adrenal (MEN-2)
    - Catecholamines (plasma and urine determinations)
- Plasma 5-HIAA
- Plasma Free metanephrines (if hypertensive)

URINE
- VMA
- Catecholamines if hypertensive or VMA is positive
- 5-HIAA (if not measured in the blood)
- 5-HTP

TISSUE IMMUNOHISTOCHEMISTRY (FORMALIN-FIXED 2-mm3 SPECIMENS): these tests are useful only to confirm a diagnosis that is based on symptoms and blood biomarker evaluations.
- CgA
- NSE
- Synaptophysin
- Ki-67, AE1, and AE3
- Glucagon
- Gastrin
- Insulin
- Somatostatin
- PP
- Consider factor VIII, CD31, and somatostatin receptors

GENETIC SCREENING
- RET protooncogene (MEN 2)
- MEN-1 gene (MEN 1)

Patient Preparation

Patient should fast overnight prior to collection of blood specimens. Antacid medications and medications affecting intestinal motility should be discontinued, if possible, for at least 48 hours prior to collection of specimens. Patients should not partake of the following foods for 48 hours prior to collection of urine for measurement of 5-HIAA and 5-HTP measurements. (*However, if the 5-HIAA plasma assay is utilized, fasting from these foods is only required for 8 hours.*)

- Cheese
- Hot dogs
- Chocolates
- Vanilla-containing foods (e.g., ice cream)
- Custard
- Pineapple, kiwi, bananas, cassava
- Avocado
- Tomato
- Walnuts

Specimen Requirements

BLOOD & URINE
See individual test listings (Chapter 4, Assays) for applicable patient preparation, specimen requirements and shipping instructions. For tests not listed, contact your contracted laboratory for applicable requirements.

TISSUE
Consult specialist for tissue staining requirements.

References
1. Please refer to Roger R. Perry in www.endotext.org/guthormones/index.htm.

©2012 Inter Science Institute. This profile for MEN syndrome screen has been copyrighted.

CPT Codes: Blood
5-HIAA (Plasma) 82542
Pituitary (MEN-1) • Prolactin 84146 • Growth Hormone 83003
Parathyroid (MEN-1 and -2) • Parathyroid Hormone (PTH) 83519 • PTHRP 83519 • Ionized Ca^{++} or Ca^{++} Corrected for Serum Albumin 82330
Pancreas (MEN-1) • Pancreatic Polypeptide 83519 • Gastrin 82938–82941 • Insulin 83525 • C-peptide 84681 • Chromogranin A 86316
Thyroid C Cells (MEN-2) • Calcitonin 82308 • Carcinoembryonic Antigen (CEA) 82378
Adrenal (MEN-2) • Catecholamines 82384
CPT Codes: Urine
Vanillyl mandelic acid (VMA) 84585
Catecholamines 82384
5-HIAA 83497
5-HTP 86316

PSEUDOGASTRINOMA SYNDROME (ATROPHIC GASTRITIS WITH LOSS OF ACID INHIBITION OF GASTRIN)

BLOOD
- Gastrin (elevated)
- Secretin stimulation test of gastrin
- Pancreastatin

If fasting gastrin level is above 100 pg/mL, order a secretin stimulation test. An increase in gastrin level greater than 100 pg/mL above the normal range denotes a gastrinoma.
- Chromogranin A (not due to a neuroendocrine tumor)
    - May be suspected with mean corpuscular volume greater than 100 μm3
- B12
- Pepsinogen I and II

Important Precaution

Patients submitted to dynamic challenge should be under the direct and constant supervision of their physician at all times. The doses listed are intended as a guideline only. The actual dose and collection schedule must be approved by the patient's physician.

Patient Preparation

Patient should fast 10 to 12 hours prior to collection of specimen. Alkali antacid medications should be discontinued, if possible, for at least 24 hours prior to collection. PPIs and H2 blockers should be discontinued for 72 hours or more prior to collection and patients monitored closely.

Specimen Collection

BLOOD & URINE
See individual test listings (Chapter 4, Assays) for applicable patient preparation, specimen requirements and shipping instructions. For tests not listed, contact your local hospital or contracted laboratory for applicable requirements.

Interpretation
Pancreastatin (collected with ISI's Z-tube™ found on page xx) plays a large role in a variety of gut-based physiological processes. Furthermore, it can serve as a useful biomarker. If a patient has elevated gastrin and CgA levels, and the presence of a normal plasma Pancreastatin level, this implies that the changes in biomarkers are from chronic PPI use or pernicious anemia, rather than the presence of a NET. Conversely, elevated CgA levels or elevated gastrin levels with elevated Pancreastatin levels should prompt clinicians to investigate the possibility of a NET.

References
1. Owyang C, Vinik AI. Diabetic pseudo Zollinger-Ellison syndrome. Gastroenterol. 1982;82(5):1144.
2. DuFour DR, Gaskin JH, Jubiz WA. Dynamic procedures in endocrinology. In: Becker KL, ed. Principles and Practice of Endocrinology and Metabolism. Philadelphia: JB Lippincott Company; 1990:1762-75.
3. Alsever RN, Gotlin RW. Handbook of Endocrine Tests in Adults and Children. Chicago: Year Book Medical Publishers, Inc.; 1978.
4. Feldman M, Schiller LR, Walsh JH, et al. Positive intravenous secretin test in patients with achlorhydria-related hypergastrinemia. Gastroenterol. 1987;93:59-62.

CPT Codes:
5-HIAA (Plasma) 82542
Gastrin 82938–82941
Chromogranin A 86316
B12 82607
Secretin Stimulation Test 82938
Pepsinogen I 83519
Pepsinogen II 83519

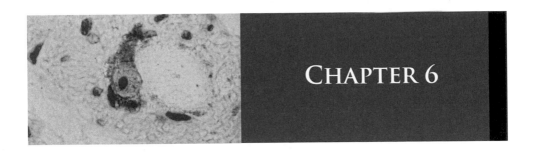

CHAPTER 6

DYNAMIC CHALLENGE PROTOCOLS, INCLUDING CPT CODES

NEUROENDOCRINE TUMORS
A COMPREHENSIVE GUIDE TO DIAGNOSIS AND MANAGEMENT

Rationale for Dynamic Challenge Protocols

Careful evaluation of GI and pancreatic disorders involves a multiplicity of interrelated factors governed by a number of hormonal axes with varying degrees of interdependence. From this composite view of interdependency, these challenge protocols are designed to help elucidate specific GI, pancreatic, and neuroendocrine abnormalities. Emphasis is placed on stimulation and/or suppression tests designed to exploit the failure of normal homeostatic regulation through metabolic pathways.

These challenge protocols represent guidelines in evaluating a variety of GI-related syndromes. The listings are selected to provide maximal information, usefulness, and significance for interpretation in the endocrine workup of the patient or research subject.

Important Notes

No patient should undergo a dynamic challenge protocol without the direct and constant supervision of trained medical personnel. The doses listed for the following protocols are intended as guidelines only. The actual dose and collection schedule must be approved by the patient's physician.

72-HOUR SUPERVISED FAST FOR THE DIAGNOSIS OF INSULINOMA

A 72-hour fast is the preferred diagnostic procedure for the diagnosis of an insulinoma.

Patient Preparation

Patient should fast for 72 hours. Water and diet soft drinks without caffeine are permitted. Patients submitted to a 72-hour fast should be under the direct and constant supervision of medical staff at all times.

Test, Times of Collection

Insulin, Glucose, C-Peptide, and Beta-Hydroxybutyrate samples are drawn at 0, 12, 24, 36, 48, and 72 hours after beginning fast. If the patient becomes symptomatic (i.e., documented fingerstick hypoglycemia) at any time during the test, blood should be drawn immediately for Insulin, Glucose, C-Peptide, and Beta-Hydroxybutyrate, unless the patient is clinically hypoglycemic. If so, delay administration of glucose until the serum glucose level is known and is >45mg/dL.

Specimen Requirements

Collect 10 mL of whole blood in a EDTA tube. Separate plasma and freeze immediately. Carefully label 3-mL EDTA tubes with time of collection and patient data.

Shipping Instructions

Specimens should be shipped frozen in dry ice.

Interpretation

Expected response in healthy people:
- Insulin levels should decrease to less than 4 μU/mL.
- Insulin/glucose ratio should be less than 0.3.

Expected response in insulinoma:
- A fasting insulin/glucose ratio greater than 0.3 is presumptive of insulinoma.
- An elevated C-peptide level greater than 4 ng/mL in the absence of obesity and insulin resistance suggests insulinoma.

Caveats

To confirm fasting, ketones should be present in the urine after 18-24 hours fasting.18-Hydroxybutyrate concentrations should also be obtained with each blood draw to support or deny suppression of insulin and release of lipolysis. Suppressed C-peptide levels (<0.5 ng/mL) during fasting suggests factitious hypoglycemia. Elevated C-peptide levels may suggest suspected sulfonylurea-induced factitious hypoglycemia and serum sulfonylurea screen should be obtained and frozen for those patients with elevated Insulin and C-Peptide levels.

References
1. Fajans SS, Vinik AI. Diagnosis and treatment of "insulinoma." In: Santen RJ, Manni A, eds. Diagnosis and Management of Endocrine-Related Tumors. Boston, MA: Martinus Nijhoff Publishers; 1984:235.
2. Vinik AI, Perry RR. Neoplasms of the gastroenteropancreatic endocrine system. In: Holland JF, Bast RC Jr, Morton DL, et al, eds. Cancer Medicine, vol. 1, 4th ed. Baltimore: Williams & Wilkins; 1997:1605-41.

CPT Codes:
C-Peptide 84681
Glucose 82947
Insulin 83525

MEAL (SHAM FEEDING) STIMULATION FOR VAGAL INTEGRITY

Test, Times of Collection

Pancreatic polypeptide: fasting; 30, 45, 60, 90, and 120 minutes after meal

Stimulus/Challenge

Following an overnight absolute fast, give patient 100 g of roast beef or other protein-rich meal or undergo sham feeding (i.e., chew food and spit out without swallowing).

Important Precautions

Patients undergoing dynamic challenge should be under the direct and constant supervision of medical staff at all times. The dosages listed are intended as a guideline only. The actual dosage and collection schedule must be approved by the patient's physician.

Specimen Requirements

Collect 3 mL serum or EDTA plasma at indicated times and separate as soon as possible. Freeze specimens immediately after separation. Minimum specimen size is 1 mL per specimen collected. Specimens should be clearly identified by time of collection.

Shipping Instructions

Specimens should be shipped frozen in dry ice.

Expected Response

Pancreatic polypeptide response should increase 2 to 5 times over baseline level.

Interpretation

Patients with impaired pancreatic function show little or no increase in pancreatic polypeptide levels. Patients with pancreatitis or diabetes mellitus often have exaggerated responses. Patients with duodenal ulcers frequently have elevated baseline levels of pancreatic polypeptide and exhibit a reduced response.

Contraindications, Interferences, Drug Effects

Patients with elevated baseline levels of pancreatic polypeptide (seen in some cases of Verner-Morrison syndrome) often have decreased responses.

References
1. DuFour DR, Gaskin JH, Jubiz WA. Dynamic procedures in endocrinology. In: Becker KL, ed. Principles and Practice of Endocrinology and Metabolism. Philadelphia, PA: JB Lippincott Company; 1990:1762-75.
2. Glaser B, Vinik AI, Sive AA, et al. Evidence for extravagal cholinergic mechanisms regulating pancreatic endocrine function. Diabetes. 1979; 28:434.

CPT Code:
Pancreatic Polypeptide 83519

ORAL GLUCOSE TOLERANCE TEST FOR DIABETES, INSULINOMA, IMPAIRED GLUCOSE TOLERANCE, METABOLIC SYNDROME, POLYCYSTIC OVARY SYNDROME (PCOS, STEIN-LEVENTHAL SYNDROME), REACTIVE HYPOGLYCEMIA, AND ACROMEGALY

Test, Times of Collection

Diabetes: measure glucose and insulin at 0 and 120 minutes. Gestational Diabetes: 0, 60, 120, and 180 minutes.

Reactive hypoglycemia: measure glucose and insulin at 0, 30, 60, 90, 120, 180, 240, and 300 minutes.

Acromegaly: measure growth hormone and glucose at 0, 30, 60, 90, 120, 180, 240, and 300 minutes.

Stimulus/Challenge

Glucose: 75 g orally

Pregnant patients: 100 g orally.

Expected Responses

Normal fasting glucose: <100 mg/dL Normal peak glucose: <200 mg/dL Normal 2 hour glucose: <140 mg/dL Impaired fasting glucose: ≥100 mg/dL

Impaired glucose tolerance (IGT or prediabetes): fasting glucose >100 mg/dL, peak >200 mg/dL and 2 hours postchallenge 141–198 mg/dL)

Diabetes: fasting glucose >125 mg/dL on 2 occasions or 2-hour glucose >200 mg/dL after oral glucose in nonpregnant patients

Reactive hypoglycemia: <40 mg/dL between 2 and 5 hours post-challenge

Normal growth hormone: <1.4 ng/mL after oral glucose

Reactive hypoglycemia: <40 mg/dL between 2 and 5 hours post-challenge

Expected Response

- Fasting insulin: 5–19 µU/mL
- Insulin should increase to at least double the baseline level and at least 10 µU/mL above baseline level
- Peak levels at 30 minutes: 50–150 µU/mL
- Return to fasting at 2 hours

A lack of a rise in serum insulin after glucose is indicative of pancreatic beta cell dysfunction. Glucose levels should be monitored to ensure validation of glucose loading. Glucose levels between 140 and 200 mg/dL indicate impaired pancreatic function. Glucose levels greater than 200 mg/dL may be indicative of diabetes. A fasting insulin/glucose ratio greater than 0.25 is presumptive for insulinoma. Proinsulin/insulin ratio greater than 0.30 is also indicative of insulinoma. Growth hormone suppresses to less than 2 ng/mL in healthy people and in patients with well-controlled acromegaly.

Insulin Resistance and Beta Cell Function

Beta cell function and insulin resistance is assessed by the HOMA model developed by Mathews using the following equations:

$$\text{HOMA IR} = \text{Fasting Insulin (µU/mL)} \times \text{Fasting Glucose (mmol/L)}/22.5$$
$$\text{HOMA B} = \text{Fasting Insulin (µU/mL)}/[\text{Fasting Glucose (mmol/L)} - 3.5]$$

Insulin secretory index is assessed by the following equation:

$$\text{Insulin secretory index} = [\text{Insulin 30 min (pmol/L)} - \text{Insulin 0 min (pmol/L)}]/$$
$$[\text{Glucose 30 min (mmol/L)} - \text{Glucose 0 min (mmol/L)}]$$

Insulin secretory index/HOMA IR ratio is used to assess insulin efficacy index.

Growth hormone levels should become undetectable within 1 to 2 hours of glucose challenge.

Important Precautions

Patients undergoing dynamic challenge should be under the direct and constant supervision of medical staff at all times. The dosages listed are intended as a guideline only. The actual dosage and collection schedule must be approved by the patient's physician.

Contraindications, Interferences, Drug Effects

Glucose levels are higher in the evening hours than in the morning hours. Glucose levels also increase with age and obesity. Pregnancy, low-carbohydrate diet, stress, contraceptives, glucocorticoids, clofibrate, thiazides, diphenylhydantoin, caffeine, ranitidine, niacin, insulin, and propanolol may increase response. Smoking, guanethidine, and salicylates may decrease response. The test should be discontinued if patient experiences vasovagal symptoms. The test should not be given to patients with glucose intolerance (i.e., those with elevated baseline glucose levels). There is also some risk of hyperosmolality.

References
1. Fajans SS, Vinik AI. Diagnosis and treatment of "insulinoma." In: Santen RJ, Manni A, eds. Diagnosis and Management of Endocrine-Related Tumors. Boston, MA: Martinus Nijhoff Publishers; 1984:235.
2. Vinik AI, Perry RR. Neoplasms of the gastroenteropancreatic endocrine system. In: Holland JF, Bast RC Jr, Morton DL, et al, eds. Cancer Medicine, vol. 1. 4th ed. Baltimore: Williams & Wilkins; 1997:1605-41.
3. American Diabetes Association. Standards of Medical Care in Diabetes. Diabetes Care. 2005;28:S4-S36.
4. Meyer CJ, Bogardus C, Mott DM, et al. The natural history of insulin secretory dysfunction and insulin resistance in the pathogenesis of type 2 diabetes mellitus. J Clin Invest. 1999;104:787-97.
5. UK Prospective Diabetes Study Group, U.K. prospective diabetes study 16: overview of 6 years' therapy of type II diabetes: a progressive disease. Diabetes. 1995;Nov;44(11):1249-58.
6. Buchanan TA, Xiang AH, Peters RK, et al. Preservation of pancreatic beta-cell function and prevention of type 2 diabetes by pharmacological treatment of insulin resistance in high-risk Hispanic women. Diabetes.2002;51:2796–803.
7. Porter LE, Freed MI, Jone NP, et al. Rosiglitazone improves beta-cell function as measured by proinsulin/insulin ratio in patients with type 2 diabetes [abstract]. Diabetes. 2000;49(Suppl 1):A122.

8. Mathews DR, Hosker JP, Rudenski AS, et al. Homeostasis model assessment: insulin resistance and beta-cell function from fasting plasma glucose and insulin concentrations in man. Diabetologia. 1985;28:412-9.
9. DuFour DR, Gaskin JH, Jubiz WA. Dynamic procedures in endocrinology. In: Becker KL, ed. Principles and Practice of Endocrinology and Metabolism. Philadelphia: JB Lippincott Company;1990:1762-75.
10. Alsever RN, Gotlin RW. Handbook of Endocrine Tests in Adults and Children. Chicago: Year Book Medical Publishers, Inc.;1978.
11. Rosenbloom AL, Wheeler L, Bianchi R. Age-adjusted analysis of insulin responses during normal and abnormal glucose tolerance tests in children and adolescents. Diabetes.1975;Sep;24(9):820-8.

CPT Codes:
Glucose Tolerance Test 82951
Glucose Tolerance Test (each additional beyond three specimens) 82952
Growth Hormone 83003
Insulin-like Growth Factor Binding Protein-3 83519
Insulin-like Growth Factor-1 84305
Insulin 83525

Pentagastrin Stimulation Test for Calcitonin (Medullary Carcinoma of the Thyroid, MCT)

The pentagastrin stimulation test is used to identify patients with MCT who have normal baseline levels of calcitonin. It is also useful to identify members of a family with a known familial form of MEN-II and MCT. Pentagastrin normally stimulates the secretion of calcitonin from the C cell. Women may not respond due to the presence of estrogens. The response in persons with MCT is an exaggeration of the normal response to pentagastrin.

Stimulus/Challenge

Pentagastrin: 0.5 μg/kg body weight by intravenous bolus injection.

CPT Code:
Calcium-Pentagastrin Stimulation 80410
Calcitonin 82308

Times of Collection

Calcitonin: 0, 1, 2, 5, and 10 minutes

Important Precautions

Patients undergoing dynamic challenge should be under the direct and constant supervision of medical staff at all times.

Specimen Collection

Collect 3 mL serum or EDTA plasma and separate as soon as possible. Freeze specimen immediately after separation. Minimum specimen size is 1 mL.

Expected Response in Patients With Medullary Carcinoma of the Thyroid

Normal basal or fasting calcitonin levels are less than 50 pg/mL. Healthy people do not experience an increase in calcitonin above 200 pg/mL with the administration of pentagastrin.

Interpretation

An exaggerated response is seen in patients with MCT and in C cell hyperplasia. Patients with elevated basal or pentagastrin-stimulated calcitonin levels should receive screening for the RET protooncogene. Carcinoembryonic antigen measurements may be helpful in determining tumor mass.

Contraindications, Interferences, Drug Effects

Patients should be warned that they will experience transient (<1–2 minutes) flushing, nausea, chest pain, and sweating with feelings (described by patients) of having impending doom after the administration of pentagastrin, but these resolve within minutes. Note: Pentagastrin remains FDA approved, but is only available from outside sources: http://www.clonagen.com/clonagen/10b2f138-2508-43df-a87e-79ec1ba77602/ pentagastrin_product.aspx.

References
1. DuFour DR, Gaskin JH, Jubiz WA. Dynamic procedures in endocrinology. In: Becker KL, ed. Principles and Practice of Endocrinology and Metabolism. Philadelphia: JB Lippincott Company; 1990:1762-75.
2. Alsever RN, Gotlin RW. Handbook of Endocrine Tests in Adults and Children.Chicago: Year Book Medical Publishers, Inc.; 1978.
3. Wells SA Jr, Baylin SB, Linehan WM, et al. Provocative agents and the diagnosis of medullary carcinoma of the thyroid gland. Ann Surg. Aug;188(2):139-41, 1978.

SECRETIN STIMULATION TEST FOR GASTRINOMA

Test, Times of Collection

Gastrin: fasting, 2, 5, 10, 15, and 30 minutes

Stimulus/Challenge

Following an overnight fast from 10:00 PM, patient should be given secretin 2 U/kg by intravenous bolus injection.

Important Precautions

Patients undergoing dynamic challenge should be under the direct and constant supervision of medical staff at all times. The doses listed are intended as a guideline only. The actual dose and collection schedule must be approved by the patient's physician.

Specimen Requirements

In adults, collect 10 mL whole blood in a EDTA tube. Separate plasma and freeze immediately. Carefully label tubes with time of collection and patient data.

Shipping Instructions

Specimens should be shipped frozen in dry ice.

Expected Response

Gastrin response should increase no more than 50% over baseline level in healthy people. In gastrinoma, the rise increase is greater than 100 pg/mL above basal levels.

Interpretation

Patients with gastrinoma exhibit elevated baseline gastrin levels and a paradoxical rise in the gastrin response to secretin greater than 100 pg/mL above the baseline level. Healthy people have a fall or no rise in gastrin levels. Patients with hypochlorhydria or achlorhydria from PPI use, type 1 gastric carcinoid, atrophic gastritis, or pernicious anemia have elevated gastrin levels (>150 pg/mL), but exhibit no response to administration of secretin. Patients with active peptic ulcers may show a 30% to 50% increase over baseline levels. Healthy patients frequently exhibit suppression in gastrin levels following secretin administration.

References
1. DuFour DR, Gaskin JH, Jubiz WA. Dynamic procedures in endocrinology. In: Becker KL, ed. Principles and Practice of Endocrinology and Metabolism. Philadelphia: JB Lippincott Company; 1990:1762-75.
2. Alsever RN, Gotlin RW. Handbook of Endocrine Tests in Adults and Children. Chicago: Year Book Medical Publishers, Inc.; 1978.
3. Feldman M, Schiller LR, Walsh JH, et al. Positive intravenous secretin test in patients with achlorhydria-related hypergastrinemia. Gastroenterology. 1987;Jul;93(1):59-62,
4. Giusti M, Sidoti M, Augeri C, et al. Effect of short-term treatment with low dosages of the proton-pump inhibitor omeprazole on serum chromogranin A levels in man. Eur J Endocrinol. 2004;Mar;150(3):299-303.

CPT Code:
Gastrin 82941
Gastrin after secretin stimulation 82938
Secretin Stimulation Test 82938

SECRETIN STIMULATION TESTING

Patient Preparation:

Nothing by mouth, except water for 12 hours before the test.

Procedure:

1. Start IV with 20 g catheter, stopcock and normal saline TKO

2. Draw one red top tube for determination of serum Gastrin levels at each of the following times:

-30 min	20 min
-15 min	30 min
0 min	60 min
3 min	90 min
5 min	120 min
10 min	

3. Secretion should be reconstituted immediately prior to use. The contents of a vial are dissolved in 8 ml of sodium Chloride Injection USP, to yield a concentration of 2 mcg/ml. Discard any unused portion after reconstitution.

4. At time 0 minutes, physician to inject the secretin IV push slowly over one minute. Usual dose is 0.4 mck/kg of body weight.

Figure 6-1. The Incretin Effect in Subjects Without and With Type 2 Diabetes

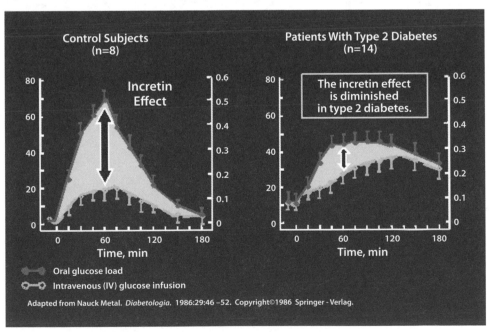

Figure 6-2. "GLP-1" Reactivity to a Glucose Meal

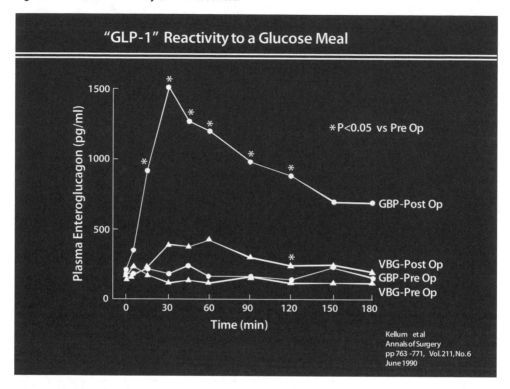

(See Chapter 4 for individual specimen collection requirements.)

CPT Code:
GLP-1 Unspecified, Immunoassay 83519
Gastrin 82941
Gastrin after secretin stimulation 82938
Secretin Stimulation Test 82938

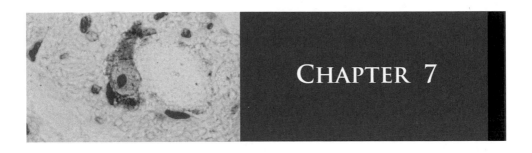

CHAPTER 7

EVALUATION AND MANAGEMENT OF NEUROENDOCRINE TUMORS

NEUROENDOCRINE TUMORS
A COMPREHENSIVE GUIDE TO DIAGNOSIS AND MANAGEMENT

ALGORITHM FOR THE EVALUATION AND MANAGEMENT OF NEUROENDOCRINE TUMORS

There are a multitude of guidelines and suggested therapeutic algorithms focused on localizing and treating NETS. Some of the more widely used guidelines include those from the ISI G.I. Council, NANETS, ENETS, and NCCN. The following guidelines are compatible with these groups' recommendations.

Modified from the NANETS Consensus Guidelines for the Diagnosis of Neuroendocrine Tumors

Aaron I. Vinik, MD, PhD, Eugene A. Woltering, MD, Richard R.P. Warner, Martyn Caplin, MD, Thomas M O'Dorisio, MD, Gregory A. Wiseman, MD, Domenico Coppola, MD, and Vay Liang W. Go, MD. Pancreas, Vol. 39(6):713-734, August 2010.

Evaluation of Neuroendocrine Tumors

Symptoms:

Clinical Syndrome

Flushing, diarrhea, wheezing, myopathy, right-sided heart disease hypoglycemia, ulcer, rash, hypertension, hyperhydrosis

Exclude other causes
Secretory vs. non secretory, wet vs. dry carcinoma, thyrotoxicosis, Cushing's, gastric bypass, medullary carcinoma of the thyroid, panic attacks, factitious symptoms

If tumor:

Biochemical and Tissue Diagnosis

Biochemical:
Plasma or Urine: 5-HIAA
Blood: serotonin, calcitonin, pancreastatin, CgA, NKA, insulin, gastrin, glucagon, PTHrp, PTH intact, Tryptase, histamine

➡ Negative ➡ **Symptomatic Treatment**

Tissue: cGA, synaptophysin, Ki-67

Figure 7-1. Most patients with NETs have a long history of vague abdominal symptoms including cramping and diarrhea with a median time from onset of symptoms to diagnosis of a NET of 9.2 years. It requires a high index of suspicion and alertness to the possibility that these symptoms are tumor

related. Flushing in NETs patients is usually dry as opposed to all other causes of flushing, which are associated with sweating. Diarrhea in a NET patient persists with fasting (ie: it is secretory). Diarrhea with gastrinoma will disappear with intake of a proton pump inhibitor. Hypoglycemia of NETs occurs for the most part with fasting and the intractable peptic ulcer disease suggests a gastrinoma. A migratory necrolytic erythema suggests a glucagonoma.

Whatever the case confirmation of the diagnosis requires a biochemical evaluation. Plasma 5-HIAA Pancreastatin, NKA, Serotonin, TCT, and tumor specific hormones such as insulin should be measured. In the absence of renal failure, hypertension or the use of a PPI, with an elevated CgA level suggests a NET. Pancrestatin is useful for prognosis as is Neurokinin A.

One should always seek confirmation with tissue histology in particular immunohistochemistry for chromogranin A, Synaptophysin and the tumor specific hormone e.g. gastrin for peptic ulcer disease. The tissue must also be stained for the marker of cell proliferation Ki-67 since this may be a determinant of choice of therapy. If all are negative, treat symptomatically and monitor at 6 month intervals to be sure there is no progression. These are slow growing tumors and should be monitored through stated biomarkers at least twice per year.

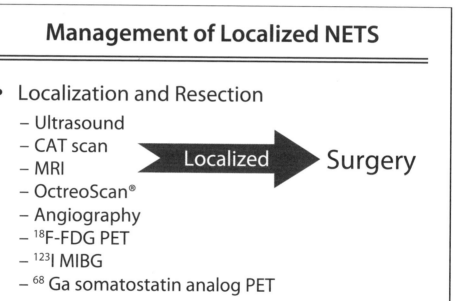

Figure 7-2. Several techniques may be required to localize a tumor including ultrasound, computerized tomography (CAT), Photon emission tomography (PET), radioactive peptide scans, such as Octreoscan and meta-iodobenzylguandine scans, as well as angiography. If localized the treatment is surgery.

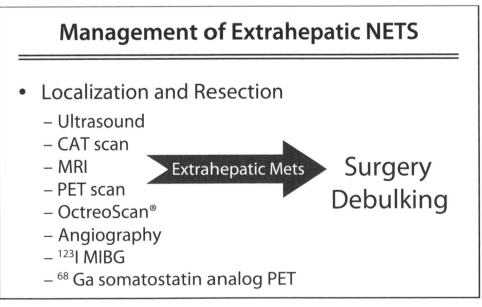

Management of Liver Predominant NETS

- Localization and Resection
  - Ultrasound
  - CAT scan
  - MRI
  - OctreoScan®
  - PET scan
  - Angiography
  - ^{123}I MIBG
  - ^{68} Ga somatostatin analog PET

Liver Involvement → Surgery

<50% RFA, Resection

>50% Partial resection, RFA, nanoknife

Therapeutic Trial

Figure 7-3. If the localization study reveals metastasis to the liver and then involvement is <50% one should attempt resection or radiofrequency ablation of the metastases. If >50% of the liver has been replaced by tumor, consider a partial resection or radiofrequency ablation, and, if possible, enter the patient into a clinical trial of current therapy.

Management of Extrahepatic NETS

- Localization and Resection
  - Ultrasound
  - CAT scan
  - MRI
  - PET scan
  - OctreoScan®
  - Angiography
  - ^{123}I MIBG
  - ^{68} Ga somatostatin analog PET

Extrahepatic Mets → Surgery Debulking

Figure 7-4. If the localization studies reveal extrahepatic metastases the aggressive surgeon may attempt surgical debulking. This may reduce tumor burden and enhance responsiveness to other medical therapies.

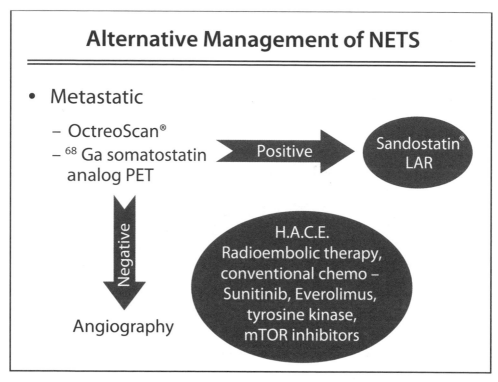

Figure 7-5. An Octreoscan is carried out. If positive, this may indicate the presence of at least somatostatin receptors 2 and 5 and implies that the tumor is likely to respond to a long acting somatostatin analog. About 40% of these patients will have escape symptoms such as diarrhea or flushing which will need rescue medication of a short acting somatostatin analog. If the Octreoscan is negative, this suggests that the tumor is devoid of somatostatin receptors and is unlikely to respond to somatostatin or its analogs. The choices are now hepatic artery chemoembolization (HACE), the use of radioactive microspheres (Radioembolic therapy), or conventional chemotherapy considering some of the newer agents, such as Sunitinib and Everolimus, tyrosine kinase and mTOR inhibitors respectively.

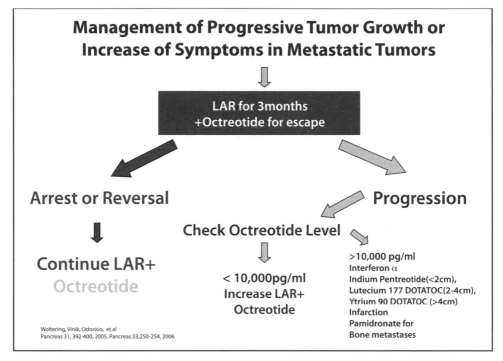

Figure 7-6. The long acting somatostatin analog (LAR or Somatuline®) should be used for 3 months and short acting analog be administered for escape from the long acting drug. If arrest or reversal of tumor growth is found continue with the Octreotide™ regime and evaluate periodically.

If the clinical response wanes or if there is tumor progression, measure the blood level of LAR and increase the dose until a circulating level of 10,000 pg/mL is found, that the receptors are saturated. If there is progression despite optimizing the circulating octreotide or Lanreotide™ levels then a trial of addition of Interferon-Alpha should be considered. If this fails, and if the tumor is <2cm, treat with Indium Pentreotide. If it is 2-4cm, the better drug is Lutecium 177 DOTATOC. Finally, if it is >4cm, Yttrium 90 DOTOTAC is the preferred treatment. Alternatively, if the tumor can be shown to have a good blood supply which is not too complicated, embolization or chemoembolization can be considered. If bone metastases are found, an infusion of pamidronate is appropriate. (Woltering, Vinik, O'Dorisio, et al. Pancreas. 2005; 31:392-400. Pancreas. 2006;33:250-254)

MEDULLARY CARCINOMA OF THE THYROID (MCT)

MCT BACKGROUND

Medullary Carcinoma of the thyroid (MCT) constitutes 2-4% of all thyroid cancer diagnoses. Biochemical diagnosis based on Calcitonin levels: 20 pg/mL as a cut-off point for basal levels with sensitivity of 100% and specificity of 93%; Calcitonin levels greater than 100 pg/mL have a positive predictive value of 100%.

Important facts:
- 25% germline RET mutation (therapeutic target)
- Somatic RET mutations in approximately 40% (worse prognosis)
- If MCT is confined to the TG, a 10-year survival occurs in >95%
- If MCT has LN involvement: 75% with distant metasases of 40%.

MCT AND GENETIC SCREENING

- All patients with (MCT) should be screened for RET gene mutations.
- Approximately 7% of apparently sporadic MCT will carry a germline RET mutation.
- RET gene screening fails in about 5% of patients.
- If no family history, the change of finding a gene mutation on repeated genetic screenings is <1%.

MCT: PREDICTING PROGRESSION

Calcitonin doubling time (DT):

Calcitonin DT (all time points)	5-year survival	10-year survival
> 2 years	100%	100%
0.5 – 2.0 years	94%	64%
<0.5 years	23%	15%

- Calcitonin <30 pg/mL before operation: all cured.
- High Ki-67 in tumor tissue

PROPOSED TESTING FOR PHEOCHROMOCYTOMAS

Pheochromocytomas are catecholamine-secreting tumors derived from chromaffin cells which are associated with sympathetic ganglia during fetal life which degenerate to leave residual cells that cluster in the adrenal medulla and some extra-adrenal sites that persist during adult life.[1,2] Between 80-85% of pheochromocytomas arise from the adrenal medulla; whereas, 15-20% arise for extra-adrenal chromaffin tissue and are known as paragangliomas[3]. Paragangliomas constitute about 30% of pediatric pheochromocytomas[4]. These occur in the carotid body, the pelvic floor and the retroperitoneum. These are exceedingly rare tumors and only account for <1% of all patients with hypertension. There are however sporadic and familial forms usually diagnosed in people aged 40-50 years; whereas, the familial forms occur in younger people. Pheochromocytomas in children are usually extra adrenal, multifocal and associated with hereditary syndromes[5].

Table 7-1. Genetic testing for Pheochromocytomas

Syndrome	Clinical Features	Chromosome	Gene
Neurofibromatosis Type 1	Multiple neurofibromas of skin and mucosae, café au lait skin and pheochromocytoma	17q11	GNDF
Von Hippel Syndrome type 1	No pheochromocytomas, renal cysts and Ca, renal and CNS hemangiomas, pancreatic neoplasms	3p25-26	VHL1
Von Hippel Syndrome type 2A	Hemangiomas, pheochromocytomas, endolymphatic sac tumors, epidermal cystadenomas		VHL2
Von Hippel Syndrome type 2B	2A +Renal cysts and carcinomas		VHL2
Von Hippel Syndrome type 2C	Pheochromocytomas only		VHL2
Paraganglioma Syndrome 1	PCs or PGLs	11q23	SDHD
Paraganglioma (PGL) Syndrome 2	PGL	11q13	Unknown
Paraganglioma Syndrome 3	PGL	1q21-23	SDHC
Paraganglioma Syndrome 4	PGL	1p36	SDHB
Carney's triad	Pheochromocytomas, gastric leimyosarcoma, pulmonary chondroma, adrenal adenoma	Unknown	Unknown
Familial PGL and gastric stromal sarcoma	PGL, gastric stromal sarcoma	Unknown	Unknown
MEN 2A	Medullary carcinoma of thyroid, pheo- chromocytomas, hyperparathyroidism, cutaneous amyloidosis	10q11.2	RET
MEN 2B	Medullary thyroid carcinoma, multiple Neuromas and marfanad habitus	10q11.2	RET

In up to 25% there may be a genetic cause. Mutations occur in the succinate dehydrogenase gene (SDH) and the SDHB mutation confers a 50% risk of metastasis.

PLASMA OR URINE METANEPHRINES AS THE BEST APPROACH FOR BIOCHEMICAL TESTING:

- **Catecholamines: non-specific, released during many conditions.**
- **Small Tumors: Catecholamines are negative.**
- **Metanephrines (NMN, MN) produced continuously and independently on catecholamine secretion.**

1st and 2nd International Symposium on PHEO (ISP) recommendations:
- **Initial testing for PHEO/PGL should include measurements of fractionated metanephrines in plasma, urine or both, as available.**
- **No consensus about plasma versus urine for preferred matrix.**

Is additional testing warranted?
- **If Free normetanephrine plasma levels are between 0.61 - 2.19 pmol/mL, further testing is needed by 20% of patients.**
- **If Free metanephrine plasma levels are between 0.31 – 1.20 pmol/mL, further testing is needed by 20% of the patients.**

Equivocal biochemical test results:
- **If results between upper reference limit (URL) and 4x above URL: use clonidine test coupled with the measurement of plasma normetanephrine (NMN, sensitivity 97%, specificity 100%)**
- **Clonidine test: distinguishes increased sympathetic activity (false positives: NMN decreases more than 40% or below URL) from PHEO/PGL (true positives).**
- **Glucagon test: if the sensitivity is less than 50%, this is not recommended.**

Imaging

Computed tomography with or without contrast can detect lesions >0.5 cm and there is no evidence that non-ionic contrast provokes a hypertensive crisis. The sensitivity (90-100%) and specificity of CT (70-80%) is comparable to that of T2-weighted magnetic resonance imaging (MRI) with gadolinium and the latter is the preferred agent. Metaiodobenzylguanidine permits the scanning of the entire body and is taken up in all chromaffin tissue and may be particularly valuable in patients in whom there is strong clinical suspicion, but not tumor is found on CT or MRI and in patients with suspect paragangliomas or extra adrenal tumors. The use of ^{131}I-MIBG may not have the sensitivity and gives poorer image quality, but more recent observations suggest that the use of ^{123}I-MIBG has a significantly greater yield and better definition of small tumors. Particularly in familial syndromes or paragangliomas this may be the tracer of choice. PET scanning using 18F-fluordopamine offers better imaging the ^{131}I-MIBG but no comparison has been made with ^{123}I-MIBG. Drugs that interfere with the recycling of catecholamines such as labetolol, calcium channel antagonists and tricyclics (TCA's) should be withheld at least 48 hours before performing the scan or a false negative can be obtained.

Management of Pheochromocytoma

The primary treatment of Pheochromocytoma is surgical extirpation laparoscopically, if possible. Patients need to be alpha adrenergically blocked and the preferred regimen is to start dibenzylline 10-14 days before surgery increasing the dose for 10 mg bid to 60 mg/day until there is complete blockade. Alpha methyl paratyrosine (metyrosine) in doses of 250 mg/day increasing to a maximum pf 2000 mg in 4 divided doses should also be given for 10-14 days. Beta blockers should only be given when complete alpha blockade has been established to prevent a hypertensive crisis due to unopposed alpha adrenergic stimulation.

Malignant Pheochromocytoma

Treatments include surgical debulking, pharmacological blockade of the adrenergic system and reduction of synthesis of catecholamines with alpha methyl paratyrosine. The use of ^{131}I-MIBG and Octreotide has not been disappointing. Combination chemotherapy with cyclophosphamide, vincristine and dacarbazine has not yielded rewarding results. The 5 year survival of malignan pheochromocytomas is about 50%[3]. There are a number of new therapies in the pipeline examining the effects of anti-angiogenic agents, inhibitors of tyrosine kinase, and the mTOR pathway and chemo-irradiation that may have greater therapeutic effectiveness. Recent evidence from Brogsitter et al shows that intraarterial infusion of ^{131}I-MIBG is more effective than systemic therapy in patients with predominant disease.

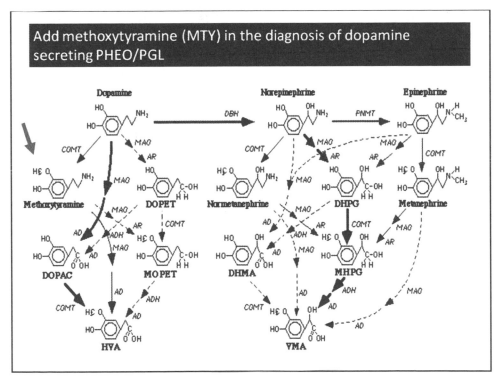

Add methoxytyramine (MTY) in the diagnosis of dopamine secreting PHEO/PGL

Figure 7-7. 3-Methoxytyramine (3-MT) is a metabolite of the neurotransmitter dopamine formed by the introduction of a methyl group to dopamine by the enzyme catechol-O-methyl transferase (COMT). 3-MT can be further metabolized by the enzyme monoamine oxidase (MAO) to form homovanillic acid (HVA), which is then typically excreted in the urine.

Eisenhower et al (Clin Chem 2011;57:411) found that 70% of SDHB/D PHEOs and 20-30% of head and neck PGLs secrete methoxytyramine (MTY), respectively.

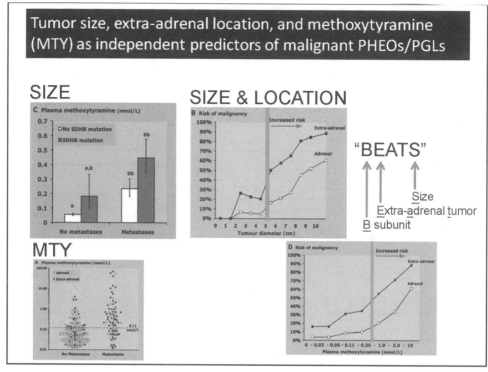

Figure 7-8. Measurement of methoxytyramine adds diagnostic and prognostic implications for patients with pheochromocytomas and paragangliomas. Elevated methoxytyramine occurs with metastases in both genetic and sporadic tumors. Plasma levels > 0.1 nmol/L suggests metastasis and a level > 0.3 nmol/L and a tumor size >5cm increases the risk of malignancy in adrenal and extra-adrenal tumors.

References:
1. Lenders et al. JAMA 2002; 287:1427
2. Banks et al. JCEM 2003; 88:553
3. Pacak et al. Nat Clin Prod Endocrinol Metab 2007;3:774
4. Eisenhower et al. JCEM 2002; 88:2658
5. Lenders et al. JCEM 2010; 95:233
6. Eisenhower et al. Clin Chem. 2011; 57:411
7. Neumann HPH, Berger DP, Sigmund G, et al. Pheochromocytomas, multiple endocrine neoplasia type 2, and von Hippel-Lindau disease. N Engl J Med 1993;329:1531-1538. [Erratum, N Engl J Med 1994;331:1535.] Eng C. The RET proto-oncogene in multiple endocrine neoplasia type 2 and Hirschsprung's disease. N Engl J Med 1996;335:943-951.
8. Gimm O, Armanios M, Dziema H, Neumann HPH, Eng C. Somatic and occult germ-line mutations in SDHD, a mitochondrial complex II gene, in non-familial pheochromocytoma. Cancer Res 2000;60:6822-6825.
9. Statement of the American Society of Clinical Oncology: genetic testing for cancer susceptibility adopted on February 20, 1996. J Clin Oncol 1996;14:1730-1736.

HOW TO AVOID CARCINOID CRISIS DURING SURGERY: GUIDELINES

- Regardless of tumor type all NETS should be pre-treated with octreotide for protection against crisis.
- Currently, studies are being performed to determine the optimal dose of octreotide to prevent Carcinoid crisis.
- Two hours prior to surgery give 500 micrograms of aqueous IV octreotide acetate followed by 100-500 micrograms per hour for the duration of the procedure.
- If the patient becomes hypotensive do not use pressors except as a last resort.
- The use of vasopressin may be helpful in patients that become hypotensive.

Two hours before surgery give 500 micrograms of octreotide acetate aqueous intravenously as an intravenous bolus. Immediately thereafter start a 500 microgram per hour IV infusion. We admix the octreotide in normal saline. We start this infusion of 500 micrograms per hour immediately after the IV octreotide push and continue the infusion during and after surgery. Depending on the severity and duration of surgery we taper the infusion over 1-24 hours. Several examples may help .For simple procedures that went smoothly such as colonoscopy we taper the infusion over 1 hour. Conversely for complex, long cases such as extensive liver resections we taper the infusion over 12-24 hours. Several warnings are in order. If the patient becomes hypotensive do not use pressors such as epinephrine, norepinephrine, or dopamine except as a last resort. To treat the hypotension use fluids and 1-5 mg bolus of octreotide (can repeat). In spite of these precautions we have had 3 cases of crisis out of approximately 500 surgical procedures. We have also seen two cases of malignant hyperthermia that occurred as part of the carcinoid crisis. We used dantrolene in normal doses along with rapid fluid administration and octreotide bolus administration and the hyperthermia responded to this treatment.

Reference:
1. Joseph S, Wang YZ, Boudreaux JP, Anthony LB, Campeaux R, Raines D, O'Dorisio TM, Go, VLW, Vinik AI, Cundiff J, Woltering EA. Neuroendocrine tumors: current recommendations for diagnosis and surgical management. Endocrinology Metabolism of North America guidelines from Clinic of North America. 2010;40:205-231.

PROPOSED TESTING FOR POST-GASTRIC BYPASS RISK FOR HYPOGLYCEMIA AND NESIDIOBLASTOSIS

Measurement of incretin effect: Insulin secretion after oral and isoglycemic intravenous glucose load.

Oral glucose tolerance tests (OGTTs) and isoglycemic intravenous glucose tests (IsoG IVGTs) were administered in the morning after a 12-hour overnight fast, on two different days, separated by <5 days.

3-hour OGTT.

All patients undergo first a 3-hour OGTT with 50 g glucose (in a total volume of 300 ml). After insertion of an intravenous (IV) catheter, at 8:00 A.M., subjects received 50 g glucose orally. Blood samples, collected in chilled EDTA tubes with added aprotinin (500 kallikrein inhibitory units/ml blood) and dipeptidyl-peptidase IV (DPPIV) inhibitor (Linco, St. Charles, MO) (10 µl/ml blood), were centrifuged at 4°C before storage at −70°C.

IsoG IVGT.

The goal of the IsoG IVGT is to expose the pancreas to blood glucose levels matched to the ones obtained during the OGTT in the same subject. Glucose (sterile 20% dextrose solution in water) is infused intravenously over 3 hours using a Gemini pump. A sample of blood is collected every 5 min using a contralateral antecubital IV catheter and then transferred in a picofuge tube without any additive and centrifuged immediately for measurement of glucose levels at the bedside. The glucose infusion rate is adjusted to match the glucose concentrations obtained for the same patient during the OGTT at each time point for 3 hours. During the OGTT and the IsoG IVGT, the arm used for blood sampling must be kept warm with a heating pad.

Incretin effect.

The difference in ß-cell responses (insulin total area under the curve [INS AUC 0–180 min]) to the oral and the isoglycemic IV glucose stimuli represents the incretin effect (INC), the action of the incretin factor expressed as the percentage of the physiological response to oral glucose, which is taken as the denominator (100%). The formula is:

$$INC = \frac{INS\ AUC_{oral} - INS\ AUC_{isoglycemic\ IV}}{INS\ AUC_{oral}} \times 100\%$$

Assays.

In the study, Total GLP-1, an indicator of secretion, was measured by radioimmunoassay (Phoenix Pharmaceutical, Belmont, CA) after plasma ethanol extraction. The intra-assay and interassay coefficients of variation (CVs) were 3–6.5 and 4.7–8.8%, respectively. This assay has 100% specificity for GLP-1, Active (7-36) and GLP-1, Inactive (9-36), 60% specificity for GLP-1, Active (7-36) and does not cross-react with glucagon (0.2%), GLP-2 (<0.001%), or exendin (<0.01%). Active GLP-1, an indicator of potential action, was measured by ELISA (Linco). The intra-assay and interassay CVs are 3–7 and 7–8%, respectively. The assay is 100% specific for GLP-1(7–36) and GLP-

1(7–37)and does not react with GLP-1(9–36), glucagon, or GLP-2. Total GIP is measured by ELISA (Linco). The assay is 100% specific for GIP 1–42 and GIP 3–42 and does not cross-react with GLP-1, GLP-2, oxyntomodulin, or glucagon. The intra-assay and interassay CVs are 3.0–8.8 and 1.8–6.1%, respectively. Plasma insulin and C-peptide concentrations are measured by radioimmunoassay (Linco) with, intra-assay CVs, respectively, of 5–8 and 3–6% and interassay CVs of 7.2 and 5.2–7.7%. The glucose concentration is measured at the bedside by the glucose oxidase method (glucose analyzer; Beckman, Fullerton, CA). All hormonal and metabolites assays performed by Inter Science Institute (ISI), Inglewood, California.

GLP-1 Meal Tolerance Test: Following a baseline blood draw, the subject is given a carbohydrate-rich, high-calorie breakfast consisting of two eggs, two strips of bacon, two pieces of whole wheat toast, and a serving of ice cream topped with flavored syrup. The test meal contains 750 kcal, 21 g of protein, 30 g of fat, and 99 g of carbohydrate. The meal should be ingested within 10 minutes to evoke the maximum response.

Timing of blood draws: Collect 5 mL of whole blood in green-topped EDTA tubes at 10, 15, 30, 45, 60, 120, and 180 minutes following completion of the meal. Glucose levels and GLP-1 should be measured. In patients with late dumping, additional blood samples should be collected after the test meal. Whole blood should be immediately separated from the frozen plasma. Specimens should be shipped frozen in dry ice.

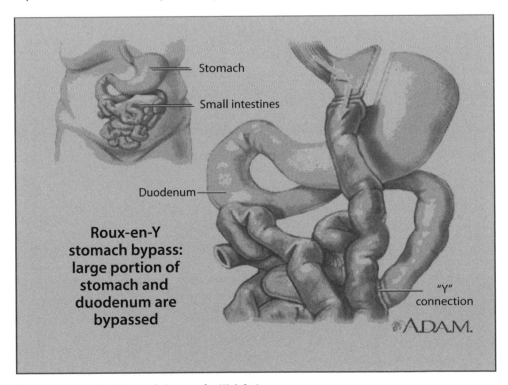

Figure 7-9. Roux-En-Y Stomach Surgery for Weight Loss

A.D.A.M., Inc. MedlinePlus Medical Encyclopedia, updated 02/04/08.

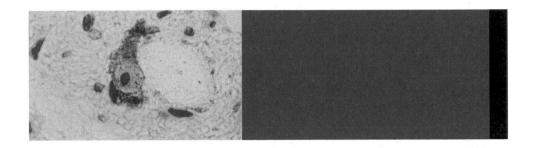

ABBREVIATIONS

ABBREVIATIONS

ACE = angiotensin-converting enzyme
ACTH = adrenocorticotropic hormone (corticotropin)
ApoE4 = apolipoprotein E4
APUD = amine precursor uptake and decarboxylation
BMI = body mass index
BNP = brain natriuretic peptide
BUN = blood urea nitrogen
CA = cancer-associated antigen
CAH = congenital adrenal hyperplasia
CCK = cholecystokinin
CEA = carcinoembryonic antigen
CgA = chromogranin A
CGRP = calcitonin gene–related peptide
CML = carboxy methyl lysine
CRH = corticotropin-releasing hormone
CRF = corticotropin-releasing factor
CRP = C-reactive protein
CSF = cerebrospinal fluid
CT = computed tomography
DDAVP = desmopressin acetate
DDI = dipsogenic diabetes insipidus
DHEA-S = dehydroepiandrosterone sulfate
DHK-PGE2 = dihydroketo prostaglandin E2
DHK-PGF2α = dihydroketo prostaglandin F2α
DIDMOAD = diabetes insipidus, diabetes mellitus, optic atrophy, and deafness
DST = dexamethasone suppression test
DVT = deep venous thrombosis
EC = enterochromaffin
ECL = enterochromaffin-like
EDTA = ethylene amine tetraacetic acid
EIA = enzyme immunoassay
EL = elastase
ELISA = enzyme-linked immunosorbent assay
FBG = fasting blood glucose
FEV1 = forced expiratory volume in 1 second
FFA = free fatty acid
FSG = fasting serum gastrin
FSH = follicle-stimulating hormone
68Ga = gadolinium-68
GAD = glutamic acid decarboxylase
GEP = gastroenteropancreatic
GEP-ET = gastroenteropancreatic endocrine tumors
GERD = gastroesophageal reflux disease
GH = growth hormone (somatotropin)
GH-RH = growth hormone–releasing hormone
GHS-R1a = growth hormone secretagogue type 1a
GI = gastrointestinal
GIP = gastric inhibitory polypeptide
GLP = glucagon-like peptide

GLP-1 = glucagon-like peptide 1
GRP = gastrin-releasing peptide
α-GSU = human glycoprotein hormone alpha subunit
5-HIAA = 5-hydroxyindoleacetic acid
5-HT = 5-hydroxytryptamine (serotonin)
5-HTP = 5-hydroxytryptophan
HDI = hypothalamic (central) diabetes insipidus
HDL = high-density lipoprotein
HLA = human leukocyte antigen
HOMA IR, B = homeostasis model assessment of insulin resistance, of beta cell function
HS CRP = highly sensitive C-reactive protein
HVA = homovanillic acid
^{123}I-MIBG = iodine-123 meta-iodobenzylguanidine
IAA = insulin autoantibodies
IAPP = islet amyloid polypeptide
IBS = irritable bowel syndrome
ICA = islet cell antigen
IgA, G = immunoglobulin A, G
IGF-1, -2 = insulin-like growth factor type 1, type 2
IGT = impaired glucose tolerance
IL-1 through IL-18 = interleukin-1 through IL-18
LAR = long-acting repeatable
LDL = low-density lipoprotein
LH = luteinizing hormone
MCT = medullary carcinoma of the thyroid
MDMA = 3,4-methylenedioxymethamphetamine
MEN-1, -2, -3 = multiple endocrine neoplasia type 1, type 2, type 3
MODY = mature-onset diabetes of youth
MRI = magnetic resonance imaging
MSH = melanocyte-stimulating hormone
MSH-α = alpha melanocyte-stimulating hormone
MSH-β = beta melanocyte-stimulating hormone
MSH-γ = gamma melanocyte-stimulating hormone
mTOR = mammalian target of rapamycin
NDI = nephrogenic diabetes insipidus
NET = neuroendocrine tumor
NETs = neuroendocrine tumors
NFκB = nuclear factor kappa B
NKA = neurokinin A
NME = necrolytic migratory erythema
NMR = nuclear magnetic resonance
NPY = neuropeptide Y
NSE = neuron-specific enolase
PAI-1 = plasminogen activator inhibitor 1
PARP = polyadenosine diphosphate ribose polymerase
PCOS = polycystic ovary syndrome
PG = prostaglandin
PG-I = pepsinogen I
PG-II = pepsinogen II
PG D2 = prostaglandin D2
PG E1 = prostaglandin E1

PG E2 = prostaglandin E2
PG F2-α = prostaglandin F2-α = prostaglandin F2-α
PHIM = peptide histidine isoleucine
pNETS = pancreatic neuroendocrine tumors
PP = pancreatic polypeptide
PPI = proton pump inhibitors
PTH = parathyroid hormone
PTHRP = parathyroid hormone–related peptide
PTHVS = percutaneous transhepatic portal, pancreatic, and hepatic venous
    gastrin sampling
PYY = peptide YY
RFA = radiofrequency ablation
SD = standard deviation
SHBG = sex hormone–binding globulin
SIADH = syndrome of inappropriate antidiuretic hormone secretion
SLI = somatostatin-like immunoreactivity
SRIF = somatotropin release–inhibiting factor
SRS = somatostatin receptor scintigraphy
T3 = triiodothyronine
T4 = thyroxine
TCT = thyrocalcitonin
THVS = transhepatic portal, pancreatic, and hepatic venous gastrin sampling
TNFα, β = tumor necrosis factor alpha, beta
TRH = thyrotropin-releasing hormone
TSH = thyroid-stimulating hormone
TTG = tissue transglutaminase
VIP = vasoactive intestinal polypeptide
VHL = von Hippel-Lindau
VMA = vanillyl mandelic acid
WDHHA = watery diarrhea syndrome (watery diarrhea, hypokalemia,
hypochlorhydria, and acidosis)
ZE = Zollinger-Ellison
ZES = Zollinger-Ellison syndrome

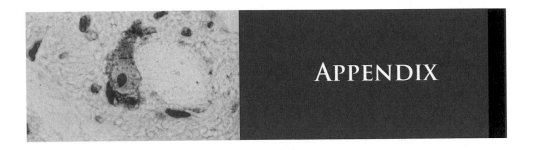

APPENDIX

WORKSHEETS

Updated with ICD-10 Codes

NEUROENDOCRINE TUMORS
A COMPREHENSIVE GUIDE TO DIAGNOSIS AND MANAGEMENT

Inter Science Institute (ISI)
944 W Hyde Park Blvd.
Inglewood CA 90302
(310) 677-3322
Fax: 677-2846

Physician, Lab, Hosp _____

Department _____

Address _____

City _____ State _____ Zip _____

Patient Name_____

Age _____ Patient Number _____

Sex _____

Specimen Type: _____

Collection Date:_____

Date Specimen
Time Rec'd at ISI: _____ AM _____ PM   ISI Accn. No.

NETs/G.I. Tests available from Inter Science Institute (ISI):

___5-HIAA (Plasma)*
___AMYLIN*
___BOMBESIN*
___C-PEPTIDE
___CALCITONIN
___CHOLECYSTOKININ (CCK)*
___CHROMOGRANIN A (CgA)
___ELASTASE
____ Serum ____ Fecal
___FREE INSULIN
___GALANIN*
___GASTRIC INHIBITORY POLYPEPTIDE (GIP)*
___GASTRIN*
___GASTRIN RELEASING PEPTIDE (GRP)*
___GHRELIN*
___GLUCAGON*
___GH-RH
___HISTAMINE
___INTERLEUKINS: _____ (1α-18)
___INSULIN
___LANREOTIDE (Somatuline Depot)
___MELANOCYTE STIMULATING HORMONE:
____α-MSH ____β-MSH ____γ-MSH
___MELATONIN ____Plasma/Serum ____Urine
___MOTILIN
___NEUROKININ A*
___NEUROPEPTIDE Y*
___NEUROTENSIN*

___OCTREOTIDE (Sandostatin®)
___PANCREASTATIN*
___PANCREATIC POLYPEPTIDE (PP)*
___PEPSINOGEN I
___PEPSINOGEN II
___PEPTIDE YY*
___PROSTAGLANDINS: PG _____
____Plasma/Serum ____Urine
___SANDOSTATIN® (Octreotide)
___SECRETIN*
___SEROTONIN (5-HT, Serum only)
___SOMATOSTATIN*
___SOMATULINE DEPOT® (Lanreotide)
___SUBSTANCE P*
___THROMBOXANE B2___Serum ___Urine
___THYROTROPIN RELEASING HORMONE*
____Plasma ____Urine
___VASOACTIVE INTESTINAL POLYPEPTIDE*
____Plasma ____Urine

PROFILES:
___BASIC NETs PROFILES:
___#100 ___#101 __-#102 ___#103
___DIARRHEA SYNDROME
___DUMPING SYNDROME
___FLUSHING SYNDROME
___SECRETIN STIMULATION

CHALLENGE PROTOCOL (Chapter 6): _____

WORKSHEET NAME (Chapter 7): _____

TOTAL VOLUME IS REQUIRED FOR URINE ASSAYS: _____ / 24 hrs.

* **ASSAYS** must be collected using ISI's specific preservative tubes **(G.I., TRH or Z-tube™)**
  Contact ISI for more information (310) 677-3322 or requests@InterScienceInstitute.com

Basic NETs Profiles available from ISI:

Neuroendocrine Tumor Profile (NET #100): for midgut patients using Octreotide
5-HIAA (Plasma)*
Pancreastatin*
Neurokinin A (NKA, Substance K)*
Substance P*
Octreotide (Sandostatin®)

Neuroendocrine Tumor Profile (NET #101):
5-HIAA (Plasma)*
Pancreastatin*
Neurokinin A (NKA, Substance K)*
Substance P

Neuroendocrine Tumor Profile (NET #102):
Pancreastatin*
Neurokinin A (NKA, Substance K)*
Substance P*
CgA (Chromogranin A)

Neuroendocrine Tumor Profile (NET #103):
Serotonin
Histamine
Substance P*
NKA (Neurokinin A)*

*Requires collection with ISI's Z-tube™ Preservative. Multiple specimens can share one 10mL Z-tube™. After collecting, separate as soon as possible. Aliquot 1mL minimum per test into separate shipping vials and freeze before shipping frozen.

[See Chapter 4 for specific patient preparation, collection requirements and shipping instructions.]

ACROMEGALY AND GIGANTISM WORKSHEET

NAME:_____   **DATE:** _____

Patient Identifier: _____   **Referring Physician:** _____

RADIOLOGY:
MRI of Sella Tercica

ROUTINE LABS:
_____CBC, CMP, Calcium ionized, GH, Lipids, Prolactin, PT, PTT, PTH, TSH

STANDARD PITUITARY LABS: SEND TO ISI (1-800-255-2873)

TEST	CPT CODES
IGF-I	84305
GH-RH (if no tumor visualized or pituitary hyperplasia on MRI)	83519
Insulin	83525

Provocative or Suppression Tests:

Oral Glucose Tolerance Test	(See Chapter 6)	82952
Somatostatin Inhibition Test	(See Chapter 6)	

TEST FREQUENCY: _____ **IMMEDIATELY**

Diagnosis:	ICD-10 CODES
Acromegaly	E22.0
Gigantism	E22.0
MEN-1	E31.21
Cushing's disease	E24.0
Cushing's syndrome	E24.9

BONE METASTASIS WORKSHEET

NAME:_____   **DATE:** _____

Patient Identifier: _____   **Referring Physician:**_____

RADIOLOGY:
____Bone Scan
Consider Octreoscan - 24 hour Planar and Spect images
Consider ^{123}I-MIBG Scan - pre-medicate with Lugol's Solution
____NO allergy to IV/Oral iodine confirmed
____Plain radiographs of weight bearing areas with bone metastasis confirmed on bone scan

---

ROUTINE LABS:
____CBC, CMP, PT, PTT
____If hypercalcemia is discovered perform 24 hour urine collection for Calcium and Phosphorus

---

STANDARD BONE METASTASIS LABS:	**CPT CODES**
____Parathyroid hormone	83970
____PTH related peptide	83519
____Alkaline phosphatase	84165
____Alkaline phosphatase isoenzymes	84080

PROVOCATIVE OR SUPRESSIVE TESTING
None recommended

Diagnosis:	**ICD-10 CODES**
Bone Metastasis	C79.51
Hypercalcemia	E83.52

NETs (Carcinoid) WORKSHEET

NAME:_____ **DATE:**_____

Patient Identifier:_____ **Referring Physician:**_____

RADIOLOGY:
____**NO allergy to IV/Oral iodine confirmed**
____**Octreoscan** - 24 planar and spect images and 48 hour planar delayed films
____**C.T. Abdomen/Pelvis** with & without IV contrast **(TRIPLE PHASE)**
____**C.T. Chest** - with & without IV contrast **(TRIPLE PHASE)**
____¹²³ **I-MIBG Scan** - pre-medicate with Lugol's Solution
____Abdominal MRI with and without Gadolinium contrast

ROUTINE LABS:
____**CBC, CMP, PT, PTT**

LABS:

BLOOD SPECIMENS TO BE SENT TO ISI:	**CPT CODES**
___Plasma 5-HIAA (Z-tube)*	82542
___CHROMOGRANIN A (Plasma or serum)	86316
___SEROTONIN (Serum only)	84260
___PANCREASTATIN (Z-tube)*	83519
___NEUROKININ A (Z-tube)*	83519
___SUBSTANCE P (Z-tube)*	83519
___Octreotide/Sandostatin® Level (Plasma or serum)	80299

(IF PATIENT ON SANDOSTATIN ONLY - Draw Immediately before next dose of Sando/LAR)

*Requires collection with ISI's special preservative tubes. Call: (800)255-2873 for supplies.

TEST FREQUENCY: _____**IMMEDIATELY** _____**3 MO** _____**6 MO** _____**1 YEAR**

SPECIMEN TO BE SENT TO YOUR REGULARLY CONTRACTED LABORATORY:
____Neuron Specific Enolase (NSE)

ICD-10 CODES **Primary site**	**Malignant**	**Benign**	**Uncert** **Behavior**	**Unspecified**
Duodenum	____C17.0	____D13.2	____D37.2	____D49.0
Lung-Bronchus	____C34.00-C34.02	____D14.30-D14.32	____D38.1	____D49.1
Stomach	____C16.9	____D13.1	____D37.1	____D49.0
Ovary	____C56.1, C56.2 or C56.9	____D27.0, D27.1 or D27.9	____D39.1	____D49.5
Thymus	____C37	____D15.0	____D38.4	____D49.89
Appendix	____C18.1	____D12.1	____D37.3	____D49.0
Colon	____C18.9	____D12.2-D12.6	____D37.8	____D49.0
Ileum	____C17.2	____D13.39	____D37.2	____D49.0
Jejunum	____C17.1	____D13.39	____D37.2	____D49.0
Rectum	____C20	____D12.8	____D37.5	____D49.0

CARCINOID SYNDROME ____E34.0

METASTATIC SITES:		
	Supraclavicular____C77.0	Retroperitoneal _____C77.2
	Brain _____C71.9	Abdominal _____C77.2
	Liver _____C78.7	Lung _____C78.00-C78.02
	Mediastinal _____C77.1	Bone _____C79.51
LIVER METASTASES	____**C7B.02**	Other_____C7B.09

DIABETES TYPE I WORKSHEET

NAME:_____   **DATE:** _____

Patient Identifier: _____   **Referring Physician:**_____

RADIOLOGY:
NONE RECOMMENDED

ROUTINE LABS:
____CBC, CMP, PT, PTT

STANDARD DIABETES TYPE I LABS:
SPECIMENS TO BE SENT TO YOUR REGULARLY CONTRACTED LAB:

	CPT CODES
____Type for HLA DR3 and DR4 genotype	86817
____Test for Islet cell antibody	86341
____Test for GAD	83519
____Test for Gastric-parietal cell	83516
____Test for Adrenal antibody	86256
____Test for Thyroid antibody	86376

SUPPRESSIVE/PROVOCATIVE TESTS
____Measure insulin secretion using fasting or arginine-stimulated C-peptide level

TEST FREQUENCY: ____**IMMEDIATELY**

ICD-10 CODES

Diabetes Type 1 (Without complication, Controlled)	E10.9
Diabetes Type 1 (Uncontrolled)	E10.65

DIABETES TYPE II WORKSHEET

NAME:_____   **DATE:** _____

Patient Identifier: _____   **Referring Physician:** _____

RADIOLOGY:
NONE RECOMMENDED

LABS:
____CBC, CMP, PT, PTT

STANDARD DIABETES TYPE II LABS:
SPECIMENS TO BE SENT TO YOUR REGULARLY CONTRACTED LAB:

	CPT CODES
____Lipoprotein profile (either VAP™or NMR method)	83704
____Triglycerides	84478
____Total Cholesterol	82465
____HDL-C	83718
____Low-density lipoprotein (LDL)-C	83721
____LDL-C particle size	83704
____Insulin	83525
____IL-6	83519
____C-peptide	80432
____C-reactive protein	86140

TEST FREQUENCY: _____**IMMEDIATELY**

ICD-10 CODES

Diabetes Type 2 (Controlled)	E11.9
Diabetes Type 2 (Uncontrolled)	E11.65

DIARRHEA SYNDROME (ICD-10 CODE: R19.7)

NAME:_____   **DATE:** _____

Patient Identifier: _____   **Referring Physician:**_____

LABS:
BLOOD SPECIMENS TO BE SENT TO ISI:

	CPT CODES
___Plasma 5-HIAA (Z-tube™)*	82542
___VASOACTIVE INTESTINAL POLYPEPTIDE (VIP) (G.I. tube)*	84586
___GASTRIN (Plasma or serum)	82941
___GASTRIN RELEASING PEPTIDE (GRP)(G.I. tube)*	83519
___PROSTAGLANDIN D2 (PG D2) (Plasma or serum)	84150
___PANCREATIC POLYPEPTIDE(Z-tube)*	83519
___CHROMOGRANIN A (Plasma or serum)	86316
___PANCREASTATIN (Z-tube™)*	83519
___SUBSTANCE P (if flushing) (Z-tube™)*	83519

*Requires collection with ISI's special preservative tubes. Call: (800)255-2873 for supplies.

SPECIMENS TO BE SENT TO YOUR REGULARLY CONTRACTED LAB:

*BLOOD SPECIMENS:*____

Calcitonin (MCT)
PTH and PTHRP if hypercalcemic
CGRP (if flushing

*URINE TESTS:*____

5-HIAA (if not collected in blood)
5-HT
VMA
CATECHOLAMINES (IF HYPERTENSIVE)

DUMPING SYNDROME WORKSHEET

NAME:_____ **DATE:** _____

Patient Identifier: _____ **Referring Physician:** _____

RADIOLOGY:
NONE RECOMMENDED

STANDARD LABS: SEND TO ISI. *Call to obtain preservative tubes: (800) 255-2873.

TEST	CPT CODES
____Insulin	83525, 80422
____Glucagon (G.I. tube)*	82943
____Pancreatic Polypeptide (PP) (Z-tube™)*	83519
____Motilin	83519
____Glucose	82947

OPTIONAL LAB:

___GLP-1, Total (G.I. tube)*	83519

SUPPRESSIVE/PROVOCATIVE TESTS

High Carbohydrate Meal
Test meal contains 750 Kcal, 21g protein, 30g fat, and 99g of carbohydrate
(2 eggs, 2 strips of bacon, a cup of decaffeinated coffee, 2 pieces of toast,
1 scoop of ice cream, and 1 ounce of chocolate syrup). The meal must be
consumed within 10 minutes. Patients with dumping syndrome usually respond
with significant rises in PP, Insulin, and Glucagon levels within 45 minutes of
ingestion of this meal. Increases in Motilin levels are usually seen 120-180
minutes after ingestion of a provocative meal.

Octreotide Suppression Meal
Measure fasting peptides, provoke with a high carbohydrate meal
Repeat on another occasion but administer 100 micrograms of Octreotide
Acetate one hour prior to meal

DIAGNOSIS:	**ICD-10 CODES**
Nonsurgical Dumping	____K30
Post Gastrectomy Dumping	____K91.1

FLUSHING SYNDROME (ICD-10 CODE: R23.2)

Tests to identify causes of flushing in different clinical syndromes.

NAME:_____   DATE: _____

Patient Identifier: _____   Referring Physician:_____

LABS:
BLOOD SPECIMENS TO BE SENT TO ISI:

	CPT CODES
___Plasma 5-HIAA (Z-tube)*	82542
___PANCREASTATIN (Z-tube)*	83519
___SUBSTANCE P (Z-tube)*	83519
___VASOACTIVE INTESTINAL POLYPEPTIDE (VIP) (G.I. tube)*	84586
___CHROMOGRANIN A (Plasma or serum)	86316
___GASTRIN (Plasma or serum)	82941
___NEUROTENSIN (Z-tube)*	83519
___HISTAMINE (EDTA Plasma only)	83008
___SEROTONIN (Serum only)	84260

*Requires collection with ISI's special preservative tubes. Call: (800)255-2873 for supplies.

SPECIMENS TO BE SENT TO YOUR REGULARLY CONTRACTED LABORATORY:

BLOOD SPECIMENS:

Calcitonin (MCT)
FSH
CGRP

URINE TESTS:

5-HIAA (if not collected in blood)
5-HT
VMA (If hypertensive)
Tryptase

GASTRIC CARCINOID WORKSHEET

NAME:_____   DATE: _____

Patient Identifier: _____   Referring Physician:_____

RADIOLOGY:
____**NO allergy to IV/Oral iodine confirmed**
____**Octreoscan** - 24 planar and spect images and 48 hour planar delayed films
____**C.T. Abdomen/Pelvis** with & without IV contrast **(TRIPLE PHASE)**
____**C.T. Chest** - with & without IV contrast **(TRIPLE PHASE)**
____ [123] **I-MIBG Scan** - pre-medicate with Lugol's Solution
____ **Abdominal MRI** with and without Gadolinium contrast.

ROUTINE LABS:
____**CBC, CMP, PT, PTT**

LABS:
BLOOD SPECIMENS TO BE SENT TO ISI:

	CPT CODES
___Plasma 5-HIAA (Z-tube)*	82542
___CHROMOGRANIN A (Plasma or serum)	86316
___SEROTONIN (Serum only)	84260
___PANCREASTATIN (Z-tube)*	83519
___NEUROKININ A (Z-tube)*	83519
___SUBSTANCE P (Z-tube)*	83519
___GHRELIN (if gastric carcinoid); (Z-tube)*	83519
___GASTRIN (Plasma or serum)	82941
___Octreotide/Sandostatin® Level (Plasma or serum)	80299

(IF PATIENT ON SANDOSTATIN ONLY: Draw immediately before next dose of Sando/LAR)
____Lanreotide/Somatuline® Depot Level (Plasma or serum)   80299
(IF PATIENT ON Somatuline® Depot ONLY: Draw immediately before next dose of SOMATULINE)

*Requires collection with ISI's special preservative tubes. Call: (800)255-2873 for supplies.

TEST FREQUENCY: _____**IMMEDIATELY** ____**3 MO** ____**6 MO** ____**1 YEAR**

SPECIMENS TO BE SENT TO YOUR REGULARLY CONTRACTED LABORATORY:

____ Neuron Specific Enolase (NSE)*	____ B-12*
____ Anti partietal cell AB*	____ Folate*
____ Anti thyroid AB*	____ Gastric pH*
____ Anti islet cell AB*	

TEST FREQUENCY: _____**IMMEDIATELY** ____**3 MO** ____**6 MO** ____**1 YEAR**

ICD-10 CODES

Primary site	Malignant	Benign
Duodenum	____C7A.010	____D3A.010
Stomach	____C7A.092	____D3A.092
CARCINOID SYNDROME	____**E34.0**	

METASTATIC SITES:

Supraclavicular	____C7B.01	Retroperitoneal	____C7B.01	Abdominal	____C7B.01
Liver	____C7B.02	Brain	____C7B.09	Mediastinal	____C7B.01
Bone	____C7B.03	Lung	____C7B.09		

GASTRINOMA INITIAL DIAGNOSIS WORKSHEET

NAME:_____   **DATE:** _____

Patient Identifier: _____   **Referring Physician:**_____

RADIOLOGY:
_____NO allergy to IV/Oral iodine confirmed
_____OctreoScan - 24 planar and spect images and 48 hour planar delayed films
_____C.T. Abdomen/Pelvis with & without IV contrast (TRIPLE PHASE)

LABS:
_____CBC, CMP, PT, PTT

GASTRINOMA LABS: CPT CODES
_____GASTRIN   82941
_____GASTRIN AFTER SECRETIN STIMULATION   82938
_____GASTRIC pH   82928

TEST FREQUENCY: _____**IMMEDIATELY**

PROVOCATIVE TESTING
SECRETIN STIMULATION TESTING (See chapter 6.)

ICD-10 CODES

Primary Site	Malignant	Benign	Uncertain Behavior	Unspecified
Ampulla	_____C24.1	_____D13.5	_____D37.6	_____D49.0
Duodenum	_____C17.0	_____D13.2	_____D37.2	_____D49.0
Jejunum	_____C17.1	_____D13.39	_____D37.2	_____D49.0
Pancreas body	_____C25.1	_____D13.6	_____D37.8	_____D49.0
Pancreas Head	_____C25.0	_____D13.6	_____D37.8	_____D49.0
Pancr Islet Cell	_____C25.4	_____D13.7	_____D37.8	_____D49.0
Pancreas Neck	_____C25.7	_____D13.6	_____D37.8	_____D49.0
Pancreas Tail	_____C25.2	_____D13.6	_____D37.8	_____D49.0
Pancreas NOS	_____C25.9	_____D13.6	_____D37.8	_____D49.0

Metastatic Sites:				
Supraclavicular	_____C77.0	Liver	_____C78.7
Abdominal	_____C77.2	Bone	_____C79.51
Mediastinal	_____C77.1	Lung	_____C78.00-C78.02
Retroperitoneal	_____C77.2	Brain	_____C71.9

Tumor classification/Syndromes:

	ICD-10 codes
MALIGNANT Neoplasm Pancreas, Produces Gastrin Islets of Langerhans	C25.4
BENIGN Neoplasm of Pancreas Produces Gastrin Islets of Langerhans	D13.7
Zollinger-Ellison Syndrome (ZES)	E16.4
MEN-1	E31.21

GHRELINOMA INITIAL DIAGNOSIS WORKSHEET

NAME:_____   **DATE:** _____

Patient Identifier: _____   **Referring Physician:** _____

RADIOLOGY:
_____NO allergy to IV/Oral iodine confirmed
_____OctreoScan - 24 planar and spect images and 48 hour planar delayed films
_____C.T. Abdomen/Pelvis with & without IV contrast (TRIPLE PHASE)

LABS:
_____CBC, CMP, PT, PTT

GREHLINOMA LABS:	**CPT CODES**
___GHRELIN (G.I. tube)*	83519
___IGF-1	84305
___CgA	86316

TEST FREQUENCY: _____IMMEDIATELY

PROVOCATIVE TESTING
NONE RECOMMENDED

ICD-10 CODES

Primary Site	Malignant	Benign	Uncertain Behavior	Unspecified
Ampulla	____C24.1	____D13.5	____D37.6	____D49.0
Duodenum	____C17.0	____D13.2	____D37.2	____D49.0
Jejunum	____C17.1	____D13.39	____D37.2	____D49.0
Pancreas body	____C25.1	____D13.6	____D37.8	____D49.0
Pancreas Head	____C25.0	____D13.6	____D37.8	____D49.0
Pancr Islet Cell	____C25.4	____D13.7	____D37.8	____D49.0
Pancreas Neck	____C25.7	____D13.6	____D37.8	____D49.0
Pancreas Tail	____C25.2	____D13.6	____D37.8	____D49.0
Pancreas NOS	____C25.9	____D13.6	____D37.8	____D49.0

Metastatic Sites:	Supraclavicular	_____C77.0	Liver	____C78.7
	Abdominal	_____C77.2	Bone	____C79.51
	Mediastinal	_____C77.1	Lung	____C78.00-C78.02
	Retroperitoneal	_____C77.2	Brain	____C71.9

Tumor classification/Syndromes:	**ICD-10 codes**
MALIGNANT Neoplasm Pancreas, Produces ghrelin Islets of Langerhans	C25.4
BENIGN Neoplasm of pancreas produces ghrelin Islets of Langerhans	D13.7

GLUCAGONOMA INITIAL DIAGNOSIS WORKSHEET

NAME:_____ **DATE:** _____

Patient Identifier: _____ **Referring Physician:** _____

RADIOLOGY:
____NO allergy to IV/Oral iodine confirmed
____OctreoScan - 24 planar and spect images and 48 hour planar delayed films
____C.T. Abdomen/Pelvis with & without IV contrast (TRIPLE PHASE)
____**Abdominal MRI** with and without Gadolinium contrast.

LABS:
____CBC, CMP, PT, PTT

LABS:
BLOOD SPECIMENS TO BE SENT TO ISI:

GLUCAGONOMA LABS:	**CPT CODES**
___GLUCAGON (G.I. tube)*	82943
___INSULIN (Plasma or serum)	83525
___ACTH (Plasma or serum)	82024
___GASTRIN (Plasma or serum)	82941
___SEROTONIN (Serum only)	84260
___VIP (G.I. tube)*	84586

*Requires collection with ISI's special preservative tubes. Call: (800)255-2873 for supplies.

SPECIMENS TO BE SENT TO YOUR REGULARLY CONTRACTED LABORATORY:
PTH
PTHRP

PROVOCATIVE TESTING
NONE RECOMMENDED

ICD-10 CODES

Primary Site	Malignant	Benign	Uncertain Behavior	Unspecified
Ampulla	____C24.1	____D13.5	____D37.6	____D49.0
Duodenum	____C17.0	____D13.2	____D37.2	____D49.0
Jejunum	____C17.1	____D13.39	____D37.2	____D49.0
Pancreas body	____C25.1	____D13.6	____D37.8	____D49.0
Pancreas Head	____C25.0	____D13.6	____D37.8	____D49.0
Pancr Islet Cell	____C25.4	____D13.7	____D37.8	____D49.0
Pancreas Neck	____C25.7	____D13.6	____D37.8	____D49.0
Pancreas Tail	____C25.2	____D13.6	____D37.8	____D49.0
Pancreas NOS	____C25.9	____D13.6	____D37.8	____D49.0

Metastatic Sites:				
Supraclavicular	____C77.0	Liver	____C78.7
Abdominal	____C77.2	Bone	____C79.51
Mediastinal	____C77.1	Lung	____C78.00-C78.02
Retroperitoneal	____C77.2	Brain	____C71.9

Tumor classification/Syndromes: **ICD-10 Codes**
MALIGNANT Neoplasm Pancreas, Produces Glucagon Islets of Langerhans   C25.4
BENIGN Neoplasm of pancreas produces glucagon Islets of Langerhans   D13.7

INSULINOMA-INITIAL DIAGNOSIS WORKSHEET

NAME:_____ **DATE:** _____

Patient Identifier: _____ **Referring Physician:** _____

RADIOLOGY:
_____NO allergy to IV/Oral iodine confirmed
_____OctreoScan - 24 planar and spect images and 48 hour planar delayed films
_____C.T. Abdomen/Pelvis with & without IV contrast (TRIPLE PHASE)
_____Abdominal MRI with and without Gadolinium contrast.

LABS:
_____CBC, CMP, PT, PTT

INSULINOMA LABS:	**CPT CODES**
____INSULIN	80422
____C-PEPTIDE	80432
____PROINSULIN	84206

TEST FREQUENCY:
_____IMMEDIATELY

PROVOCATIVE TESTING
A 72-HOUR SUPERVISED FAST WITH INSULIN/ C-PEPTIDE/GLUCOSE LEVELS STAT WHEN PATIENT
BECOMES SYMPTOMATIC.

ICD-10 CODES Primary Site	Malignant	Benign	Uncertain Behavior	Unspecified
Ampulla	____C24.1	____D13.5	____D37.6	____D49.0
Duodenum	____C17.0	____D13.2	____D37.2	____D49.0
Jejunum	____C17.1	____D13.39	____D37.2	____D49.0
Pancreas body	____C25.1	____D13.6	____D37.8	____D49.0
Pancreas Head	____C25.0	____D13.6	____D37.8	____D49.0
Pancr Islet Cell	____C25.4	____D13.7	____D37.8	____D49.0
Pancreas Neck	____C25.7	____D13.6	____D37.8	____D49.0
Pancreas Tail	____C25.2	____D13.6	____D37.8	____D49.0
Pancreas NOS	____C25.9	____D13.6	____D37.8	____D49.0

Metastatic Sites:					
Supraclavicular	_____C77.0		Liver	____C78.7
Abdominal	_____C77.2		Bone	____C79.51
Mediastinal	_____C77.1		Lung	____C78.00-C78.02
Retroperitoneal	_____C77.2		Brain	____C71.9

Tumor classification/Syndromes:	**ICD-10 Codes**
MALIGNANT Neoplasm Pancreas produces Insulin Islets of Langerhans	C25.4
BENIGN Neoplasm of pancreas Islets of Langerhans	D13.7
MEN-I	E31.21

PNET (ISLET CELL) DIAGNOSIS WORKSHEET

NAME:_____ **DATE:** _____

Patient Identifier: _____ **Referring Physician:**_____

RADIOLOGY:
____**NO allergy to IV/Oral iodine confirmed**
____**OctreoScan - 24** planar and spect images and 48 hour planar delayed films
____**C.T. Abdomen/Pelvis with & without IV contrast (TRIPLE PHASE)**
____**C.T. Chest - with & without contrast (TRIPLE PHASE)**
____**MRI with Gadolinium contrast liver/pancreas only**

LABS:
____**CBC, CMP, Calcitonin, PT, PTT, PTH intact**

LABS:
BLOOD SPECIMENS TO BE SENT TO ISI:

pNET LABS:	**CPT Codes**
____Growth Hormone (Plasma or serum)	83003
____Glucagon (G.I. tube)*	82943
____Gastrin (Plasma or serum)	83519
____Ghrelin (G.I. tube)*	83519
____Somatostatin (G.I. tube)*	84307
____Insulin (Plasma or serum)	83525
____C-Peptide (Plasma or serum)	84681
____Pancreatic Polypeptide (Z-tube)*	83519
____Motilin (Plasma or serum)	83519
____Vasoactive Intestinal Polypeptide (VIP) (G.I. tube)*	84586
____Insulin Like Growth Factor 1 (G.I. tube)*	83519
____Octreotide/Sandostatin Level (If patient is on Sandostatin only)	80299
____Lanreotide Level (If patient is on Somatuline® Depot only)	80299

*Requires collection with ISI's special preservative tubes. Call: (800)255-2873 for supplies.

TEST FREQUENCY: _____**IMMEDIATELY** ____**3 MO** ____**6 MO** ____ **1 YEAR**

ICD-10 CODES

Primary Site	Malignant	Benign	Uncertain Behavior	Unspecified
Ampulla	____C24.1	____D13.5	____D37.6	____D49.0
Duodenum	____C17.0	____D13.2	____D37.2	____D49.0
Jejunum	____C17.1	____D13.39	____D37.2	____D49.0
Pancreas body	____C25.1	____D13.6	____D37.8	____D49.0
Pancreas Head	____C25.0	____D13.6	____D37.8	____D49.0
Pancr Islet Cell	____C25.4	____D13.7	____D37.8	____D49.0
Pancreas Neck	____C25.7	____D13.6	____D37.8	____D49.0
Pancreas Tail	____C25.2	____D13.6	____D37.8	____D49.0
Pancreas NOS	____C25.9	____D13.6	____D37.8	____D49.0

Metastatic Sites:

Supraclavicular	_____C77.0	Liver	____C78.7
Abdominal	_____C77.2	Bone	____C79.51
Mediastinal	_____C77.1	Lung	____C78.00-C78.02
Retroperitoneal	_____C77.2	Brain	____C71.9

Syndromes: MALIGNANT Neoplasm Pancreas, Producing Insulin, Somatostatin or Glucagon

Islets of Langerhans	____C25.4
ZOLLINGER-ELLISON SYNDROME	____E16.4
WHIPPLE'S DISEASE	____K90.81
SWEET'S DISEASE	____L98.2
MEN-I	____E31.21

MEN-1 INITIAL DIAGNOSIS WORKSHEET

NAME:_____   **DATE:** _____

Patient Identifier: _____   **Referring Physician:**_____

RADIOLOGY:
____NO allergy to IV/Oral iodine confirmed
____OctreoScan - 24 planar and spect images and 48 hour planar delayed films
____C.T. Abdomen/Pelvis with & without IV contrast (TRIPLE PHASE)
____Sestimibi scan for parathyroid
____MRI of pituitary
____**Abdominal MRI** with and without Gadolinium contrast.

LABS:
FASTING CBC, CMP, Calcium, Calcium Ionized, Calcium-Phosphorous, Prolactin

---

MEN-1LABS:	**CPT CODES**
___GASTRIN (Plasma or serum)	82941
___GASTRIN AFTER SECRETIN STIMULATION (Plasma or serum)	82938
___GASTRIC pH	82928
___INSULIN (Plasma or serum)	83525
___C-PEPTIDE (Plasma or serum)	84681
___PARATHYROID (INTACT)	83970
___GROWTH HORMONE (Plasma or serum)	83003

TEST FREQUENCY:
_____**IMMEDIATELY**

PROVOCATIVE TESTING
SECRETIN STIMULATION TESTING FOR GASTRINOMA (See chapter 6.)
72 HOUR SUPERVISED FAST FOR INSULINOMA (See chapter 6.)

SUPRESSIVE TESTS
OCTREOTIDE SUPRESSION TEST

ICD-10 CODES

Primary Site	Malignant	Benign	Uncertain Behavior	Unspecified
Ampulla	____C24.1	____D13.5	____D37.6	____D49.0
Duodenum	____C17.0	____D13.2	____D37.2	____D49.0
Jejunum	____C17.1	____D13.39	____D37.2	____D49.0
Pancreas body	____C25.1	____D13.6	____D37.8	____D49.0
Pancreas Head	____C25.0	____D13.6	____D37.8	____D49.0
Pancr Islet Cell	____C25.4	____D13.7	____D37.8	____D49.0
Pancreas Neck	____C25.7	____D13.6	____D37.8	____D49.0
Pancreas Tail	____C25.2	____D13.6	____D37.8	____D49.0
Pancreas NOS	____C25.9	____D13.6	____D37.8	____D49.0
Parathyroid	____C75.0	____D35.1	____D44.2	____D49.7
Pituitary	____C75.1	____D35.2	____D44.3	____D49.7

Metastatic Sites:

Supraclavicular	____C77.0	Liver	____C78.7
Abdominal	____C77.2	Bone	____C79.51
Mediastinal	____C77.1	Lung	____C78.00-C78.02
Retroperitoneal	____C77.2	Brain	____C71.9

Associated Tumors and Syndromes	ICD-10 Codes
MALIGNANT Neoplasm Pancreas, Produces Insulin Islets of Langerhans	C25.4
BENIGN Neoplasm of Pancreas Produces Insulin Islets of Langerhans	D13.7
MALIGNANT Neoplasm Pancreas, Produces Gastrin Islets of Langerhans	C25.4
BENIGN Neoplasm of Pancreas Produces Gastrin Islets of Langerhans	D13.7
Parathyroid	D35.1
Pituitary	D35.2
MEN-I	E31.21
Zollinger Ellison Syndrome	F16.4

MEN-II INITIAL DIAGNOSIS WORKSHEET

NAME:_____ **DATE:** _____

Patient Identifier: _____ **Referring Physician:**_____

RADIOLOGY:
____NO allergy to IV/Oral iodine confirmed
____OctreoScan - 24 planar and spect images and 48 hour planar delayed films
____C.T. Abdomen/Pelvis with & without IV contrast (TRIPLE PHASE)
____Sestimibi scan for parathyroid
____MRI of pituitary
____**Abdominal MRI** with and without Gadolinium contrast.

ROUTINE LABS:	**CPT CODES**
FASTING CBC, CMP,	82310
CALCIUM	82330
CALCIUM IONIZED	
24 HOUR URINE FOR CALCIUM-PHOSPHOROUS	
VMA	

MEN-2 LABS:	**CPT CODES**
CALCITONIN	82308
PARATHYROID (INTACT)	83970
CATECHOLAMINES TOTAL URINE	82383
CATECHOLAMINES BLOOD	82383
CATECHOLAMINES FRACTIONATED	82384
PLASMA FREE METANEPHERINES	86316

TEST FREQUENCY:
_____IMMEDIATELY

PROVOCATIVE/SUPRESSIVE TESTING
See supressive and provocative testing for pheochromocytoma (page 207-211).
See provocative testing for Medullary Carcinoma of thyroid with pentagastrin (page 199).

ICD-10 CODES

Primary Site	Malignant	Benign	Uncertain behavior
Adrenal	____C74.9	____D35.0	____D44.1
Parathyroid	____C74.90-C74.92	____C35.00-D35.02	____C44.10-D44.12
Pituitary	____C75.1	____D35.2	____D44.3
Thyroid	____C73	____D34	____D44.0

Associated Tumors and Syndromes	**ICD-10 Codes**
Hyperparathyroidism	E21.3
Disorder of calcitonin secretion	E07.0
Secretion of catecholamines by pheochromocytoma	E27.5

MEDULLARY CARCINOMA OF THE THYROID INITIAL DIAGNOSIS WORKSHEET

NAME:_____ DATE: _____

Patient Identifier: _____ Referring Physician: _____

RADIOLOGY:
CONSIDER CT SCAN OF NECK
CONSIDER METASTATIC WORK UP

LABS:
____CBC, CMP, PT, PTT, Carcinoembryonic Antigen (CEA)

MCT LABS:		**CPT CODE**
CALCITONIN		82308
CONSIDER GENETIC TESTING FOR MCT	HC PCS	53840

TEST FREQUENCY:
_____**IMMEDIATELY**

PROVOCATIVE/SUPRESSIVE TESTING
NONE: PENTAGASTRIN STMULATION IS NO LONGER USED

	ICD-10 CODES
MALIGNANT NEOPLASM OF THYROID	C73
HYPERSECRETION OF CALCITONIN	E07.0
MEN-2A	E31.22
MEN-2B	E31.23

PANCREATIC POLYPEPTIDE (PP-OMA) INITIAL DIAGNOSIS WORKSHEET

NAME: _____ **DATE:** _____

Patient Identifier: _____ **Referring Physician:** _____

RADIOLOGY:
_____NO allergy to IV/Oral iodine confirmed
_____OctreoScan - 24 planar and spect images and 48 hour planar delayed films
_____C.T. Abdomen/Pelvis with & without IV contrast (TRIPLE PHASE)
_____**Abdominal MRI** with and without Gadolinium contrast.

LABS:
_____CBC, CMP, PT, PTT

LABS:
BLOOD SPECIMENS TO BE SENT TO ISI:

PP-oma LABS:	**CPT CODE**
_____PANCREATIC POLYPEPTIDE (Z-tube)*	83519

*Requires collection with ISI's special preservative tubes. Call: (800)255-2873 for supplies.

TEST FREQUENCY:
_____IMMEDIATELY

PROVOCATIVE TESTING
NONE RECOMMENDED

ICD-10 CODES

Primary Site	Malignant	Benign	Uncertain Behavior	Unspecified
Ampulla	_____C24.1	_____D13.5	_____D37.6	_____D49.0
Duodenum	_____C17.0	_____D13.2	_____D37.2	_____D49.0
Jejunum	_____C17.1	_____D13.39	_____D37.2	_____D49.0
Pancreas body	_____C25.1	_____D13.6	_____D37.8	_____D49.0
Pancreas Head	_____C25.0	_____D13.6	_____D37.8	_____D49.0
Pancr Islet Cell	_____C25.4	_____D13.7	_____D37.8	_____D49.0
Pancreas Neck	_____C25.7	_____D13.6	_____D37.8	_____D49.0
Pancreas Tail	_____C25.2	_____D13.6	_____D37.8	_____D49.0
Pancreas NOS	_____C25.9	_____D13.6	_____D37.8	_____D49.0

Metastatic Sites:	Supraclavicular	_____C77.0	Liver	_____C78.7
	Abdominal	_____C77.2	Bone	_____C79.51
	Mediastinal	_____C77.1	Lung	_____C78.00-C78.02

Tumor classification/Syndromes:	**ICD-10 CODES**
MALIGNANT Neoplasm Pancreas, (Produces Pancreatic Polypeptide Islets of Langerhans)	C25.4
BENIGN Neoplasm Pancreas, (Produces Pancreatic Polypeptide Islets of Langerhans)	D13.7

PHEOCHROMOCYTOMA WORKSHEET

NAME:_____   DATE: _____

Patient Identifier: _____   Referring Physician: _____

RADIOLOGY
____**T2 weighted MRI from neck to the bladder**
____ [123] **I-MIBG Scan** - pre-medicate with Lugol's Solution
____**Consider** [111] **In pentetreotide scan (OctreoScan®)**

LABS:
BLOOD SPECIMENS TO BE SENT TO ISI:

PHEOCHROMOCYTOMA LABS:	CPT CODES
____Pancreastatin (Z-tube)*	83519
____Chromogranin A (CgA) (Plasma or serum)	86316

*Requires collection with ISI's special preservative tubes. Call: (800)255-2873 for supplies.

SPECIMENS TO BE SENT TO YOUR REGULARLY CONTRACTED LABORATORY:
____Plasma Free Metanephrines
____24 hour urine for VMA, metanephrine, normetanephrine, epinephrine, norepinephrine
____Plasma for metanephrine, normetanephrine, epinephrine, norepinephrine, dopamine

---

INTERPRETATION OF LAB VALUES:
If plasma metanephrine is 4x above the upper reference limit (URL) a Pheochromocytoma is biochemically proven. It is then appropriate to move to radiologic for localization. If plasma metanephrine value is between URL and 4x above the URL, a Clonidine test with the measurement of plasma free normetanephrine can be used. The elevation of only dopamine can reflect SDHB-related (familial) Pheochromocytoma.

TO PERFORM A CLONIDINE SUPPRESSION TEST:
Clonidine suppression test=0.3mg per 70KG. Draw labs at 0 min and 3 hours after Clonidine administration. If normetanephrine is below 40% of baseline or if below URL - the diagnosis of Pheochromocytoma is NOT supported.

ICD-10 CODES:

Primary Site Pheochromocytoma	Malignant	Benign	Uncertain Behavior	Unspecified
Unspecified site	____D49.7	____D35.9	____D44.9	____D49.0
Adrenal neoplasm	____C74.90-C74.92	____D35.00	____D44.10	____D49.7
Neoplasm of bladder				____D49.4
Neoplasm of sympathetic nervous system				____D49.7
Hypertension				____I15.8
Medullary hyperfunction				
Hypersecretion of catecholamines by pheochromocytoma				____E27.5

UNKNOWN OR NON-FUNCTIONAL NET INITIAL DIAGNOSIS WORKSHEET

NAME:_____ **DATE:** _____

Patient Identifier: _____ **Referring Physician:**_____

RADIOLOGY:
_____NO allergy to IV/Oral iodine confirmed
_____OctreoScan - 24 planar and spect images and 48 hour planar delayed films
_____C.T. Abdomen/Pelvis with & without IV contrast (TRIPLE PHASE)
_____MRI abdomen with Gadolinium contrast-Liver pancreas only

---

LABS:
_____CBC, CMP, PT, PTT

LABS:
BLOOD SPECIMENS TO BE SENT TO ISI:

NON-FUNCTIONAL OR UNKNOWN NET LABS:	CPT CODES
___Plasma 5-HIAA (Z-tube)*	82542
___PANCREATIC POLYPEPTIDE (PP) (Z-tube)*	83519
___CHROMOGRANIN A (Plasma or serum)	34468
___PANCREASTATIN (Z-tube)*	83519
___GLUCAGON (G.I. tube)*	82943
___INSULIN (Plasma or serum)	83525
___ACTH (Plasma or serum)	82024
___SUBSTANCE P (Z-tube)*	84801
___GASTRIN (Plasma or serum)	83519
___SEROTONIN (Serum only)	84260
___VASOACTIVE INTESTINAL POLYPEPTIDE (VIP) (G.I. tube)*	84686
___GHRELIN (G.I. tube)*	83519

*Requires collection with ISI's special preservative tubes. Call: (800)255-2873 for supplies.

ICD-10 CODES

Primary Site	Malignant	Benign	Uncertain Behavior	Unspecified
Ampulla	_____C24.1	_____D13.5	_____D37.6	_____D49.0
Duodenum	_____C17.0	_____D13.2	_____D37.2	_____D49.0
Jejunum	_____C17.1	_____D13.39	_____D37.2	_____D49.0
Pancreas body	_____C25.1	_____D13.6	_____D37.8	_____D49.0
Pancreas Head	_____C25.0	_____D13.6	_____D37.8	_____D49.0
Pancr Islet Cell	_____C25.4	_____D13.7	_____D37.8	_____D49.0
Pancreas Neck	_____C25.7	_____D13.6	_____D37.8	_____D49.0
Pancreas Tail	_____C25.2	_____D13.6	_____D37.8	_____D49.0
Pancreas NOS	_____C25.9	_____D13.6	_____D37.8	_____D49.0

Metastatic Sites:	Supraclavicular	_____C77.0	Liver	_____C78.7
	Abdominal	_____C77.2	Bone	_____C79.51
	Mediastinal	_____C77.1	Lung	_____C78.00-C78.02
	Retroperitoneal	_____C77.2	Brain	_____C71.9

Tumor classification/Syndromes:	**ICD-10 Codes**
MALIGNANT Neoplasm Pancreas, Produces pancreatic polypeptide Islets of Langerhans	C25.4
BENIGN Neoplasm of pancreas produces pancreatic polypeptide Islets of Langerhans	D13.7

PRIMARY HYPERPARATHYROIDISM
INITIAL DIAGNOSIS WORKSHEET

NAME:_____   **DATE:** _____

Patient Identifier: _____   **Referring Physician:**_____

RADIOLOGY:
_____SESTIMIBI SCAN
_____Ultrasound Parathyroid/neck

LABS:
_____CBC, CMP, PT, PTT, Calcium, Calcium ionized

PARATHYROID LABS:	**CPT CODES**
INTACT PTH	83970
24 HOUR URINE FOR CALCIUM AND PHOSPHORUS	81099
PTHrP IN PATEINTS WITH KNOWN MALIGNANCY	

TEST FREQUENCY: _____**IMMEDIATELY**

PROVOCATIVE/SUPRESSIVE TESTING	**CPT CODE**
DIET CONTROLLED 24 HR URINE CALCIUM COLLECTIONS	81099

	ICD-10 CODES
Primary Hyperparathyroidism	E21.0
Secondary hyperparathyroidism due to renal disease	N25.81
Secondary hyperparathyroidism (non-renal)	E21.1
Tertiary hyperparathyroidism	E21.2
MEN-1	E31.21
MEN-2A	E31.22
MEN-2B	E31.23

SOMATOSTATINOMA INITIAL DIAGNOSIS WORKSHEET

NAME:_____ **DATE:** _____

Patient Identifier: _____ **Referring Physician:** _____

RADIOLOGY:
_____NO allergy to IV/Oral iodine confirmed
_____OctreoScan - 24 planar and spect images and 48 hour planar delayed films
_____C.T. Abdomen/Pelvis with & without IV contrast (TRIPLE PHASE)
_____Abdominal MRI with and without Gadolinium contrast.

LABS:
_____CBC, CMP, PT, PTT

LABS:
BLOOD SPECIMENS TO BE SENT TO ISI:

SOMATOSTATINOMA LABS:	CPT CODE
SOMATOSTATIN (G.I. tube)*	84307

*Requires collection with ISI's special preservative tube. Call: (800)255-2873 for supplies.

TEST FREQUENCY:
_____**IMMEDIATELY**

PROVOCATIVE TESTING
NONE RECOMMENDED

ICD-10 CODES

Primary Site	Malignant	Benign	Uncertain Behavior	Unspecified
Ampulla	_____C24.1	_____D13.5	_____D37.6	_____D49.0
Duodenum	_____C17.0	_____D13.2	_____D37.2	_____D49.0
Jejunum	_____C17.1	_____D13.39	_____D37.2	_____D49.0
Pancreas body	_____C25.1	_____D13.6	_____D37.8	_____D49.0
Pancreas Head	_____C25.0	_____D13.6	_____D37.8	_____D49.0
Pancr Islet Cell	_____C25.4	_____D13.7	_____D37.8	_____D49.0
Pancreas Neck	_____C25.7	_____D13.6	_____D37.8	_____D49.0
Pancreas Tail	_____C25.2	_____D13.6	_____D37.8	_____D49.0
Pancreas NOS	_____C25.9	_____D13.6	_____D37.8	_____D49.0

Metastatic Sites:

Supraclavicular	_____C77.0	Liver	_____C78.7
Abdominal	_____C77.2	Bone	_____C79.51
Mediastinal	_____C77.1	Lung	_____C78.00-C78.02
Retroperitoneal	_____C77.2	Brain	_____C71.9

Tumor classification/Syndromes:	ICD-10 Codes
MALIGNANT Neoplasm Pancreas, Produces somatostatin Islets of Langerhans	C25.4
BENIGN Neoplasm of pancreas Produces somatostatin Islets of Langerhans	D13.7

VIPOMA INITIAL DIAGNOSIS WORKSHEET

NAME:_____   **DATE:** _____

Patient Identifier: _____   **Referring Physician:** _____

RADIOLOGY:
_____NO allergy to IV/Oral iodine confirmed
_____OctreoScan - 24 planar and spect images and 48 hour planar delayed films
_____C.T. Abdomen/Pelvis with & without IV contrast (TRIPLE PHASE)
_____Abdominal MRI with and without Gadolinium contrast

LABS:
____CBC, CMP, PT, PTT

LABS:
BLOOD SPECIMEN TO BE SENT TO ISI:

VIPOMA LABS:	**CPT CODES**
____VASOACTIVE INTESTINAL POLYPEPTIDE (VIP) (G.I. tube)*	84586

*Requires collection with ISI's special G.I. preservative tube. Call: (800)255-2873 for supplies.

SPECIMENS TO BE SENT TO YOUR REGULARLY CONTRACTED LABORATORY:
STOOL pH & Gastric pH

TEST FREQUENCY: _____IMMEDIATELY

PROVOCATIVE TESTING
NONE RECOMMENDED

ICD-10 CODES

Primary Site	Malignant	Benign	Uncertain Behavior	Unspecified
Ampulla	____C24.1	____D13.5	____D37.6	____D49.0
Duodenum	____C17.0	____D13.2	____D37.2	____D49.0
Jejunum	____C17.1	____D13.39	____D37.2	____D49.0
Pancreas body	____C25.1	____D13.6	____D37.8	____D49.0
Pancreas Head	____C25.0	____D13.6	____D37.8	____D49.0
Pancr Islet Cell	____C25.4	____D13.7	____D37.8	____D49.0
Pancreas Neck	____C25.7	____D13.6	____D37.8	____D49.0
Pancreas Tail	____C25.2	____D13.6	____D37.8	____D49.0
Pancreas NOS	____C25.9	____D13.6	____D37.8	____D49.0

Metastatic Sites:	Supraclavicular	_____C77.0	Liver	____C78.7
	Abdominal	_____C77.2	Bone	____C79.51
	Mediastinal	_____C77.1	Lung	____C78.00-C78.02
	Retroperitoneal	_____C77.2	Brain	____C71.9

Tumor classification/Syndromes:	**ICD-10 Codes**
MALIGNANT Neoplasm Pancreas, Produces VIP Islets of Langerhans	C25.4
BENIGN Neoplasm of pancreas produces VIP Islets of Langerhans	D13.7

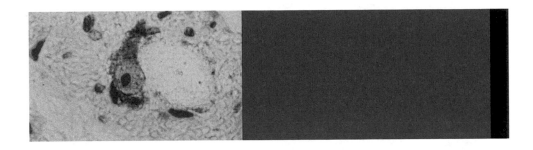

INDEX

I